I was wearing a dress I hadn't worn in ages and summer sandals for the tropical heat. "You look so good," one of the moms commented. Normally, I would be so excited with this ego-boosting compliment. But she had no idea I lost so much weight because I had been sick - the irony was thick because I had been trying my whole adult life to slim down. She also didn't know how happy I was to overcome my weakness and be able to walk from the car park to the school. There were other things she wasn't aware of either: how much I was sweating because I was so out of shape from all the time spent lying in bed, or how long it took me to shower and dress because of the unbearably painful hemorrhoids. My mind was thinking, "Don't you know I have cancer?" But all I said was "Thank you."

—∞—

I started telling people that getting a cancer diagnosis was the "kick in the pants" I needed to focus on true health. I didn't think of myself as a naughty disciple, but more of an adult experiencing light bulb clarities, and forced to learn more about life and myself. This gave me an opportunity to dig deeper, look within myself, understand my psyche, be able to hold tight and let go, and learn to be vulnerable. I was given a chance to grow, a chance to question, a chance to sit still, a chance to listen, and a chance to change.

"*Finding My Healthy* was written with a passion for helping women who have faced the cancer diagnosis; with hope and practical solutions. It is filled with stories of Gina's own journey and how she was able to move through her illness and find a healthy balance in her life. I would recommend this book to anyone who is facing cancer; is a post cancer patient, or someone who is sharing a cancer patient's journey."

Caterina Barregar, The Empowerment Diva
North America's Relationship and Worthiness Coach
www.caterinabarregar.com

finding
MY
healthy

a TRUE STORY of THRIVING after CANCER

Gina Twellmann

finding MY *healthy*

ISBN-13: 978-0-9970968-9-7
ISBN-10: 0-9970968-9-6

Published by: Celebrity Expert Author
http://celebrityexpertauthor.com

Canadian Address:
501- 1155 The High Street,
Coquitlam, BC, Canada
V3B.7W4
Phone: (604) 941-3041
Fax: (604) 944-7993

US Address:
1300 Boblett Street
Unit A-218
Blaine, WA 98230
Phone: (866) 492-6623
Fax: (250) 493-6603

Medical Disclaimer

The information provided in this book is designed to provide helpful information on the subjects discussed. This book is not intended as a substitute for the medical advice of physicians. For diagnosis or treatment of any medical problem, the reader should regularly consult a physician in matters relating to his/her health and particularly with respect to any symptoms that may require diagnosis or medical attention. The publisher and author are not responsible for any specific health or allergy needs that may require medical supervision and are not liable for any damages or negative consequences from any treatment, action, application or preparation, to any person reading or following the information in this book. References are provided for informational purposes only and do not constitute endorsement of any websites or other sources.

Cover design by Umbrella² Design Group
Cover photography by LinQreative
Original poetry by Gina Twellmann

And the day came when the risk to remain tight in a bud was more painful than the risk it took to blossom.

~ Anais Nin

Contents

Intro

I am a Gemini, which often gives me an excuse for the contradictions. But everyone has a journey of ups and downs. Sometimes I am focused, feeling above the daily issues and craving a better version of myself. On those days I want to eat clean, be connected to my food choices, and find health so that I can reach my potential of being authentic. Other times, I want out of my journey; I find the moment difficult, and I use refined sugars to escape from my perception of stress.

I've been in remission and cancer free since July 2014 and have learned a lot in the process — in fact, I am still learning. My type of cancer diagnosis was different as well, and considered rare but also very receptive to treatment. I like to think that the combination of all my detoxing and efforts, in addition to the chemo and other targeted therapy meds, had worked well together. One of the difficult aspects of dealing with cancer is that western medicine and alternative research are frequently at odds with each other — the former tells us to "do this and act quick," while the latter urges us not to listen to traditional doctors and do something totally different. The two sides don't seem to meet in the middle very often, leaving us, the patients, to decide ourselves what to do while feeling unwell and pressured by those around us to choose the best care. So don't be afraid to step back and slow down the process. Be comfortable every step of the way, listen to your voice, your heart, the universe, God — whatever leads you in a direction of feeling light and easy and true.

There are so many people who joined me on the journey to health, helping me to get out of my own way and hear the things I already knew in my heart. Through motivation, fitness, support, nutrition, and healing, I am so grateful to have met them: Nathalie Tellier, Corinne Mackay, Robert Kirby, Sharlene Morgante, Jacqueline Graham, Eric Standop, and Dr. Gregory Cheng.

Chapter 1.
How did I get to this point?

I was having such a good week. I had been going to boot camp classes, boxing fitness or Pilates every weekday. Mind you, I was feeling faint several times whenever I pushed myself but kept thinking I was having blood sugar or blood pressure issues. I still wanted to lose weight, even though in the last year I had already lost 40 pounds! I lived in Macau (an autonomous region on the south coast of China) with my husband, Paddy, and twin toddlers, a boy and a girl. I was a teacher at an International School, living the expat life, always meeting new people. But feeling a bit burned out, I had stopped working the previous summer, wanting to spend time getting fit after gaining too much weight after the kids were born.

I had always struggled with weight. Back in high school, my first boyfriend had a slim build and was also shorter than me. No matter how much affection and loving looks I got, a small part of me kept thinking I needed to stay slim. I ran several mornings a week and made sure I signed up for an early morning gym class since I was already so busy with music practice and homework later in the day. Groceries were shared among seven people in the house so there weren't many extra snacks. But I was so hungry after morning band practice that I often ate half of my lunch before school had even started, leaving me with little for the rest of the day and no snack money for the cafeteria cookies and French fries.

When university started, I signed up for a food plan that was included with my dorm fees. You could choose A, B, or C plans, depending on how much you thought you would eat or use the cafeteria. I think I chose the B plan. It was so convenient: every time I went for a meal, all I had to do was swipe a card. I didn't have to look at grocery fliers, plan a menu, or go shopping for the week. This was supposed to leave me free to study, which sounded good in theory, but it also made it way too easy to get all the treats and choices I had never had on a daily basis. Whenever it was crunch time for a 5000-word paper or a final exam, it was easy to find someone who wanted to walk over to the evening café to meet the temptation of coffees, cookies, muffins, and other quick treats. The food was a cheap way to release some stress since all I had to do was swipe a card. So it wasn't long before I had gained 20 pounds. And once I was teaching, I became so concentrated on doing well that balance went out the window. There was always something to prepare, cut, make, or research when creating lesson plans. At the start of my teaching career, I really didn't have a sense of myself, which resulted in a lot of stress. After a day spent with so many little personalities needing my attention, I just wanted to unwind. Having a chocolate bar or a bowl of cereal was a relaxing and cheap indulgence, and I gained another 20 pounds.

For the next few years, I was on and off diets. I continued working and ended up in Korea, Taiwan, and finally Macao (close to Hong Kong). I was running occasionally and thought I was fit, not noticing how out of shape I really was. In between the bouts of fitness, there was a lot of alcohol and rich food. I had a long pregnancy with twins and a 12- week bed rest that resulted in a lot of muscle loss. I thought I had recovered well, doing Pilates to regain some core strength so I could get up and down from the floor and pick up those babies! But a year before my diagnosis, work was leaving me stressed and I decided I needed a change. Paddy supported my decision and I stopped work with the intention of taking a year to get healthy.

Q. Have you ever kept up with the demands of work and family while ignoring your own health?

I was not squandering my time and the workouts had become my morning routine. I found a great training group that I had heard about years before but had never been energetic enough to get up early enough for those morning boot camp classes. Now that I wasn't working, and the kids had preschool classes in the morning, I could easily get the exercise.

Losing weight became my new focus and I signed up for lots of classes. My trainer had such variety – alternating among obstacle courses, rotating stations, kettlebells, cardio boxing and even my least favorite – sprint training. I started wearing a Jawbone band to track my fitness and my sleep. It's amazing how addictive this band can be. I didn't want to exercise without it but then the sweating started to break it; the boxing gloves didn't really work with it either, but it was great to track my fitness. I was so obsessed to see the record of my sleep progress that when the band stopped working one day, I couldn't help moaning, "But how will I know how

I slept?" And the great part of exercising in Macau is that we were outside all the time; in tropical climates, the more you sweat, the more you feel like you're really working out.

I had stopped work in June and even during Christmas 2013 I was still going strong — my Type A personality was in full gear and I wasn't going to fail. We rented a house for Christmas, which meant we could decide how many treats we brought in. I felt in control of my goals. I wasn't really thinking about detox; I just wanted to maintain my exercise to lose the weight. By January, I felt I had reached one goal: I had lost 30 pounds! Many years ago, Paddy had made a bet with me that if I got to a specific weight, he would stop smoking. Either he thought it was a safe bet I wouldn't lose the weight or he needed an outside push to get him to quit. At the time, I believed I could easily win but life got in the way and I never seemed to make this goal a priority long enough to make a difference. But by the end of January 2014, I had finally won the bet. True to his words, my husband stopped smoking and I was released of the little voice in the back of my head that would remind me of how guilty I would have felt if I hadn't lost the weight and he hadn't stopped smoking and had gotten sick because of it. I knew it was his choice, but the voice was there anyway. I think I even announced something on Facebook so there was some celebrating and I felt like a fit person. Sometimes when you change gradually, it takes others to remind you of the progress you've made. One day my trainer and a friend reminded me that my clothes were looser now and that yes, there was a visible difference. It took a while to register. Then one day, my trainer surprised me with a gift of crop fit training gear from the store where I didn't think I could fit anything! And they fit! I was so motivated by the new size and I think my trainer was tired of seeing me in the same long training pants when it was getting hotter and hotter outside. I was running more now and became interested in trail hikers and trail running. It was a great feeling to be navigating a trail path, adjusting to the landscape, earphones on and enjoying the challenge of the moment while also being able to push myself.

Q. When has the way others see you not matched the way you see yourself?

The only problem was I often fell asleep after lunch. But it seemed understandable because I often got up at 5:30 am for the 6 am boot camp class, then came home for a quick shower, got dressed while my husband made the kids breakfast, and I took them to school. Then I would be on my second pair of workout clothes, ready to rush to the 8:45 am class that was often a repeat of the earlier one. It was kind of fun - several of the moms at the International School had free time in the morning and so many of them were off to do some kind of workout — whether it was cross-fit, a walk up on the hill, Pilates, or Yoga. Now that I was getting fitter, I didn't mind being seen dropping off my kids in my training gear. By the time the morning workout was done and I had had a shower, it was almost time for lunch. A nap following lunch became a habit and almost necessary to get on with the day. I thought I was just tired from all the exercise. Other times, I would squeeze in a late afternoon cardio boxing class before dinner. I had a helper/nanny so it wasn't too hard to leave for an hour. Often, near the end of the class, there would be some core work on the mats after all the cardio boxing. I was pushing myself so hard. I remember commenting to my training partner or the trainer that I felt faint, or that my ears were ringing. But I attributed these symptoms to blood pressure or blood sugar problems, never suspecting anything else and neither did anyone else.

Then it was the first week of March 2014. On a Wednesday evening, Paddy and I went to the symphony. We hadn't gone in ages and we both had fun. The next morning I started getting a migraine. This often happened during hormonal cycles so I didn't give it much attention. I was pretty much guaranteed one migraine a month just before my period, especially if I had already worked out and had muscle tension or was tired. I have a picture from the evening we went to the symphony. I often look at it to see if I could notice anything different. In addition to a migraine, the twins were home sick battling coughs so I didn't have much time to rest. They ended up staying home again on Friday, so there was still no time for rest. I had to cancel my evening plans with my husband. While trying to relieve an unending migraine with some pain pills, I briefly noticed that I could hear a noise in my lungs while breathing. But I wasn't coughing, so I kept plowing through Saturday, getting up early with the kids, not realizing how sick I already was. Those migraine pills have a bit of codeine in them, which allowed me to cope, without being really aware of everything that was happening around me. This was a first — I had never before had a migraine last more than one day!

Finally, on Sunday morning my daughter was feeling better but I decided I had better try to get some treatment for my son's cough or his teacher wouldn't like me too much Monday morning. Since I also wasn't feeling better, I rounded up the whole family and we begrudgingly headed off to the clinic, hoping it wouldn't take too long and we could go back to a restful Sunday. I went to one doctor first; by then, I was probably on the third day of my chest crackling but since I wasn't coughing, I didn't think to bring it up to the doctor. So he hadn't listened to my chest or given me antibiotics, just a bunch of pills — one of them was to keep me from getting nauseous from so many medications! Although I had great treatments from Chinese doctors while in Southeast Asia, I am sorry to say this was typical of what I had experienced from Western medicine in Taiwan and Macau so far. Feeling like I was wasting our Sunday, I stuffed the bags of pills into my purse and rounded up the family to head over to the clinic next door for the kids, at which point I realized how late it was and sent Paddy off with my daughter to get some snacks. Due to the many days of dealing with a migraine, I hadn't eaten very much and was feeling quite weak. Just as my husband and daughter returned, I suddenly announced, "I'm going to faint," and my poor son must have gotten quite a shock as he was sitting on my lap at the time.

A bit of advice here: never faint in a hospital! I remember fainting once before. I was in Taiwan on my own, struggling with being sick and having to work. I went to the doctor and received a shot of antibiotics and then he sent me on my way. No one suggested I might need to rest a bit first as the shot might make me feel sick. I went off on my 125cc "scooter" and after a few minutes, things started going white. I kept blinking my eyes but it didn't help and the next thing I knew I was sitting on the side of the road, my scooter lying beside me with the engine still running. I was trying to process what had just happened. Now, as then, I was also trying to process what was happening. I woke up in a wheelchair being pushed towards an emergency room. I couldn't figure out where my family was and what was going on.

This was the start a series of confusing hospital events, to say the least. Keep in mind that I was in Macau, speaking to doctors and nurses to whom English was a second language so good communication wasn't easy. While several doctors were trying to assess my situation, one emergency care physician said he thought I had had an ectopic pregnancy and I tried to explain that he was totally off base as I had just started my period. Another doctor said that I'd lost too much blood. I couldn't understand what he was talking about. I tried to convince them that I was faint from the migraine and lack of food the last few days, so would they please let me go as my kids were sick and I had to take them home to make lunch! I felt like I was losing control of the situation and was getting anxious to tell my children that Mommy was okay. Then the doctor started using scare tactics and convinced my husband that I needed to go to the main hospital to get checked out. Paddy started saying that he would call our helper (it was her day off) to come and watch the kids. We had never called her on a Sunday and it all sounded very dramatic to me. I regretted going to the clinic that morning and wished I could turn back the clock. My husband told me the doctors reacted quickly and had been doing tests for the past hour but lying on the examining table, I seemed to have no say in the situation. The next thing I knew I was in the ambulance on the way to the main hospital.

Q. Have there been moments when you've been sick and felt you lacked control of the type of treatment given to you?

My husband arrived at the general hospital after sorting a sitter for the kids. The doctors told me I needed a blood transfusion, as my red cells were too low. I signed the papers to agree but then realized that the transfusion would take about four to six hours and we had plans for the Rolling Stones concert that evening! Everyone in town had been talking about this event and I had already canceled other plans that weekend. I wasn't going to miss the concert. I convinced the doctors to let me go but once we got home and I started getting ready, I realized I was too ill to go anywhere. While I stayed in bed, Paddy rushed off an hour before the concert to find someone who would buy our tickets. Looking back, it's crazy to think that I already had double pneumonia by this point (plus cancer), which none of the three doctors at the two hospitals I visited in the last 24 hours had noticed.

I spent the night in the reclining chair, as it was the only way I could breathe, but I still didn't put two and two together. By the morning I was getting anxious, as I couldn't even will myself to get up and walk across the living room to get some water. I became scared and told Paddy I had to go to the hospital again. He asked our friends in a flat below to come up and watch the kids and I was off in an ambulance by 7 am. As I was being wheel-chaired out of the house, my husband told the kids to say bye to Mommy but they sat watching TV and wouldn't even turn their heads.

I thought that getting to Emergency early on a Monday morning, when everyone was going to work or school, would mean a quick diagnosis and care, and being back home before lunch. As it turned out, I was so wrong. My husband dropped me off and was going to check in at work while I got examined. Hours later, I was still lying on a stretcher in the hallway, being moved from hallways to rooms, next to a variety of seniors with an assortment of aches and pains. They seemed to be either moaning or chatting away while food and bedpans were exchanged. It was a sickie party and I couldn't stand it. I had blood tests, an ultrasound, x-rays, and my hospital bed kept getting parked in different places. No one talked to me (because of the language barrier?) and it was all I could do to get someone's attention to beg for some water. Thank goodness I didn't need to use the washroom. I wasn't going to be part of the bedpan party. Later in the afternoon, my husband returned and a Portuguese doctor came and talked to us. (Macao used to be a Portuguese colony so the main languages are Cantonese and Portuguese.)

He told us I had double pneumonia and was very anemic. I was close to a 90% oxygen saturation level, which is a borderline limit for needing oxygen, and he recommended that I check in for an overnight stay. Somehow, discussing my x-ray results while hanging out in a hospital bed in the hallway didn't make things feel very urgent. I protested a bit but finally agreed to a night in the hospital. Luckily, my oxygen tank and antibiotic drip were mobile and I could still get to the bathroom. The nurse asked me to take a sleeping pill and I obliged, hoping a night of rest would do me good. I shared a room with two other ladies. I respected them as elderly women and I had no idea why they were hospitalized, but I quickly realized that the sleeping pill would be of no help against the noise of my roommates. The maddening clang of machines was also disturbing me. One lady slept-talked in Cantonese and the nurses shouted throughout the night. It was horrible.

The next morning, the nurses woke me up at 6:30 am to request more tests and give me some food that was a mush of something I can hardly remember. I had to get out. How could I listen to my breathing and meditate on healthy lungs with all the chaos around me? I needed to be surrounded by my own things. The nurse said I had to wait until the doctors came, around four hours later. Three of them stood at the foot of my bed, urging me to stay in the hospital. I felt like they were ganging up on me, saying there was something wrong with my blood. I tried my best to look well and thought how hard it was to fight for oneself when one is sick. I could hear an eager curiosity in their voices as they were trying to figure out my case but I thought, never mind my blood, let me fix my lungs first so I could breathe.

Several hours later, and with great reservations from both the doctors and my husband, I was let out. Paddy became my reluctant nursemaid: checking fevers, tracking my food intake, monitoring my antibiotics, and helping me shower. On the evening of the day I was released from the hospital, one doctor phoned Paddy, telling him I should come back to the hospital. He suspected I had Hairy Cell Leukemia. I thought he was over-reacting but, as it turned out, he was right.

Chapter 2.

What happens when you have a fever for four weeks?

Two weeks later, I already had one blood transfusion but was still close to fainting. My husband did not like it that I had discharged myself from the hospital. Because of double pneumonia, I could barely breathe and the constant fever clouded my brain. I had antibiotics and fever medication. I just read a study from the University of Alberta that recommended not allowing pneumonia patients with less than 92% oxygen saturation to be outpatients. Maybe that is a good approach. Paddy never gets ill and was not prepared to be a nursemaid, but he ended up in that role anyway. I guess I looked sick enough that he didn't think I could make good decisions on my own and he was worried I wouldn't take the antibiotics. So he took the control and rationed out the meds throughout the day, starting to record every time I ate or drank something, while also recording my temperature. It all seemed very clinical to me but I was too ill to respond. Besides the night sweats and dizziness, I was in a mental state, where people seemed to move either too fast or too slow and everything happened outside the bubble of my sickness. I hadn't been as ill since suffering from pneumonia the age of 10, but even then I remember everything seeming so surreal that I couldn't engage in any activity while dinner preparations were going on. This is how I felt again now. The first couple of weeks I couldn't take care of my kids at all. I didn't know what was happening in the outside world; all I could feel was how sick I was.

I knew that the doctor had mentioned Hairy Cell Leukemia and a problem with my blood but this diagnosis was really not even in my range of thinking yet. For a while, I couldn't really grasp a possible cancer diagnosis. I knew that my pneumonia was bad, and after having just been at a boot camp and the symphony concert the week before, I couldn't understand how or why my immune system weakened so suddenly. Whenever I got sick in the past, my mind automatically started figuring out what I had done wrong to get ill. This time was the same but I only had a moment to reflect on the how and the why – I just couldn't think clearly!

Q. Have you ever been so sick that you felt you were losing control of regaining health?

I remember the time when my grandmother was in the hospital just before she passed away. Mormor had always been healthy and strong. She had been taking care of herself for many years on her own, not spending much time talking about the aches and pains of aging. But when she had fallen and hurt her hip, all of a sudden she was in the hospital. I was so far away that I couldn't see her and assess her state of mind. Our brief phone conversation made me think she was thinking about the past and not looking toward the future anymore. It was bittersweet and on some level, I was angry – wishing she would fight a bit more. She was in pain but in my mind, she was giving up. Yet, with my continuing fever, sweats, fainting episodes, and lack of energy to barely get out of bed, I started to have some empathy for my grandmother. I think there comes a point, especially once you start having more painkiller medication, that you really can't focus anymore — never mind having to conjure up a will to fight against pain and suffering. It might not even be a choice to let go… after some time in this state; the body and the mind just can't handle any more stress. Previously, I had always believed that the mind could conquer illness if you reach for the internal motivation and will to recover – now I wasn't so sure.

I lay in bed, trying to think about what I should eat to stay healthy, even though I didn't feel like eating. Paddy thought I wasn't taking in enough nutrition, so he even started writing down my meals. Small bowls of food would arrive by my bedside and my instinct told me to only eat the most nutritious, whole foods, without any additives or sugar. I'd have a small bowl of berries for breakfast, some broth or chicken soup for lunch, and a few bites of rice with frozen peas for dinner. My lovely friend started bringing some food – amazing soup, rich in greens. It wasn't a lot of calories but I had extra pounds to spare anyway. I kept drinking lots of water and gave my body the rest it was shouting out for. I didn't like all the antibiotics but I had no choice with the constant fever that would rise throughout the day. The fever lasted a month and gave me the by-product of a kick-started detox. I also thought a lot about my breathing. Looking back, I wonder if all the time I spent staring out the window not thinking about anything could be considered as effective as hours of meditation.

I found something similar to Pranayama breathing on the Internet and started using this technique to build up my oxygen. In Sanskrit, Pranayama means "extension of the prana or life force" or "breath control." In Yoga practice, the idea is that control and extension of the breath can manipulate your energy to soothe your mind. But I found an article that used the breathing technique to actually build up oxygen supply. It was something like breathe in for four counts, hold for two, and breathe out for four counts. Regardless of the technique, slowing down and focusing my breathing undoubtedly brought oxygen into my cells and lungs. I couldn't sleep all day but I couldn't do anything either, so I had time to breathe. Paddy had gone out and bought an oxygen saturation tester, which measured my resting heart rate and oxygen saturation from a finger pulse. I had to make sure it didn't go down to 90% or I would have to go back to the hospital.

My condition prevented me from taking care of my kids, but I already had a helper for about six hours a day. In Macau, the helpers coming to work from the Philippines were part maids, part housecleaners, and part babysitters. We had had Faye working for us since the twins were two weeks old and she was a great help. At least I didn't have to worry about cleaning the house and my husband paid the bills. What I couldn't let go of was the need to know what my children were doing. Paddy would make breakfast and get the kids ready for school. He was perfectly capable of this task but I was the one who usually reminded the kids when it was library day, what they should wear for the weather, or to not forget their water bottles and please brush their hair. The daily routine was usually my job and many times when I couldn't get out of bed, I shouted orders and reminders from the bedroom, trying to micromanage the household and solve conflicts when I heard the twins bugging each other. It sounds silly now, but being a mother is not a job you can delegate, no matter how sick you are. I had to learn to let go. A network of moms and families who were happy to help surrounded us, but I had never needed to ask for help, having developed a sense of independence while living overseas. As expats, we were used to dealing with and solving problems on our own, because communication and cultural differences in our host countries were not always easy. Being so ill made it necessary for me to ask other moms to drive my kids home from school and my helper could then greet them on our street.

Q. How much do you trust your own advice, your doctor's diagnosis, or your friends' and family's suggestions?

While I was busy asking other moms for help with my children, my husband was busy looking for a doctor. We didn't really trust the government hospital. We had heard too many stories of misdiagnoses: one teacher at school was told she most likely had a brain tumor, while it turned out to be just a bump on the head. Another expat was diagnosed with a possible tumor, but the tumor seen in the scan was actually her uterus! We even opted to have the twins born in a private Hong Kong hospital, not trusting the local hospital to handle a caesarean or that my husband would be allowed near the babies if they ended up in ICU for a while. Through our running group, we realized that one of our friends was a doctor! (Usually, we were busy running and socializing and not talking about work and what people did for a living). Paddy contacted her and asked her to come by the house.

I put on a brave face, determined that she wouldn't suggest to Paddy that I go back to the hospital. If you've ever had a few too many drinks, you might relate to the feeling of thinking you're fooling everyone and believing that everyone thinks you're sober. And then someone tells you the next day what you were saying and you realize you weren't fooling anyone. That's probably what happened when our doctor friend came to visit. It was in the evening, so my fever was already getting higher and I was trying not to look sweaty. I told her I was aware of my breathing, hydration, eating quality foods (although not very much) and taking all my meds, but I think I probably looked very pale and glassy-eyed. She said I was doing the right things, reassured my husband, and recommended someone we could see. He was a consultant from Hong Kong who was working at the University Hospital in town. This was perfect, as I didn't have the energy to hop on a plane to Canada or catch a ferry to Hong Kong. We were so relieved to find a specialist in blood cancers.

I went to the hospital to have a bone marrow extraction. The attending nurses were so lovely. I tried to put on a brave face but finally had to admit that after having to get dressed, get in the car, and sit in the waiting chair, I was close to fainting again. The doctor's ferry was late so the nurses suggested I go to sleep in one of the diagnostic room beds. I was so thankful to be horizontal again and just focused on breathing. A bone marrow extraction is not fun and quite painful, especially if they don't get enough of a sample the first time. But it didn't take long. The marrow extraction was going to be sent to Hong Kong for examination and diagnosis, which would either confirm or exclude Hairy Cell Leukemia, but the blood test already said a lot. My platelets were low, causing lots of bruising (which I thought was from the kids always banging into me!); my hemoglobin was low as well (explaining all the fainting); and my white cells were also too low, explaining the sudden onset of double pneumonia. There was also my spleen; I already knew from the ultrasound the day after I fainted that my spleen was enlarged.

Hairy Cell Leukemia (HCL) sounded so odd; I had to get straight on the Internet to try to figure it out for myself. Having information was subconsciously my way of feeling in control of the situation. I didn't realize there were so many types of leukemia. I had an image of a patient with pale skin that is weak and needs a bone marrow transplant to survive. But there are over a dozen different types of this illness, either slow growing and chronic or fast developing and acute. HCL, first identified in 1958, is a former kind — a slow-growing blood cancer where the bone marrow makes too many B cells (lymphocytes). I had to look it up and I needed to understand more. All blood cells start as stem cells and they divide up to create different white blood cells (including lymphocytes) that fight infection, red blood cells that carry oxygen to the body, and platelets that are important in blood clotting. The B lymphocyte cells in patients with HCL are abnormal and under a microscope, they look like they have lines coming out from them, hence the name Hairy Cell. These cells overcrowd the other cells, resulting in low red cells and platelets. The abnormal cells can also build up in the spleen or liver. HCL is very rare, usually affecting more men than women, and usually older than middle-aged adults, so I was clearly an anomaly. A UK cancer research site indicates that of the 8,300 cases of leukemia diagnosed each year, only 220 cases are HCL. In the United States, about three cases out of every million are HCL, and about 800-900 new cases are diagnosed each year.

My husband kept a dutiful set of notes to help him feel in control of the chaos I had brought into the household. I moved into the guest bedroom and I started a new routine of dealing with double pneumonia and the effects of leukemia — a routine that included fever medicine, antibiotics, cough medicine, sleeping, and a bit of food. A few hours later and I'd start the rotation over again, several times a day, waiting for my husband and helper to bring me water, help me get dressed, and bring the kids to visit with me. After a month, my lungs cleared themselves, the fever lifted, and I was off the antibiotics. Now I had to deal with the underlying diagnosis – cancer.

Chapter 3.
How can I detox?

I live in a town of expats with a network of many acquaintances and friends. I also have family and friends spread around the world. I thought the easiest method of getting the word of my diagnosis out there was to post it on Facebook and tell everyone at the same time. How exhausting this process turned out to be! After putting up a post, it took me three hours of texting to respond to all the messages. Since I was overseas, it was easier to text but it wasn't less tiring since I was repeating the same information to people asking questions about what had happened. In a way, I felt I — the sick one — was taking on a strange role of comforting *them* – making sure they knew I was okay and that I had a plan. I felt guilty if I didn't respond, thinking that, if I didn't put their minds at ease, I was contributing to *their* stress. A couple of times I said to family members, "I can't talk now – I can't breathe." It wasn't their fault. How would they know how much I was suffering if I didn't tell them? You don't get much information from a text.

There was also a lot of disbelief about my diagnosis. People knew I was suffering from pneumonia but didn't realize how sick I really was. Most urged me to get second opinions, to not trust the doctors in our area, and then wished me well. As I mentioned before, there had been several misdiagnosis stories circulating around the expat community from the past. Patients were often given the worst possible case scenario first so that the doctor could change the diagnosis to better news after further investigation. That is why when I went to the hospital for a blood transfusion; I became quite agitated when the nurses kept referring to me as the leukemia patient. At the time, no diagnosis had yet been established and I didn't completely trust the nurses at the university hospital. In my mind, they were just in training.

Obviously, I had a lot to process. When I was a young teen, I often had the thought pop into my head that I was going to catch a disease and die prematurely. I was a bit of a dramatic philosopher in my teenage years but I don't really know where this thought came from. So when I heard the HCL diagnosis, I thought, "Oh no, I was right!" The next thought was probably the first of many stages in dealing with the news – the disbelief. I had quit work the year before to get healthy, had lost weight and was stronger than ever, working out five times a week. In Dr. J.C. Holland's book, *The Human Side of Cancer*, she suggests that disbelief is a protective device from the psyche so that there is time to let the information sink in and not get overwhelmed at the start. The second stage is the turmoil phase where, as reality is confronted, one alternates between fear and calm, and there is a preoccupation with the diagnosis.[1]

I wanted help but I wasn't prepared for the barrage of advice people were giving me —even though it was undoubtedly well

---

1   Holland, J. C. & S. Lewis, *The Human Side of Cancer: Living with Hope, Coping with Uncertainty* (Quill: New York, 2000) p. 45.

intentioned. I welcomed the suggestions, but I was nervous to try things when I was already so sick. For example, one friend messaged me that her friend had cured leukemia with Guanabana, a fruit found in Africa, South America and Southeast Asia and also known as a sour sop, Graviola, and Brazilian paw-paw. But I hardly had the energy to look this up. When you have so many contradictory messages on websites, it's not easy to decide what's good for you. While one site warned against using the extract of sour sop, referencing a 1997 study that had showed better results in treating breast cancer than chemotherapy, there were no clinical trials to prove the results, and other sites warned that the toxicity of the extract could lead to Parkinson's disease. Another site claimed that sour sop was 10,000 times more effective than chemotherapy and it was only because the drug companies couldn't replicate the extract that it hadn't been advertised well. Looking back, I still am not sure how to process all this data, but it probably wouldn't have hurt me to have eaten some of the fruit, in less concentrated forms. At the time, however, I was too sick to do all the necessary research and I didn't have access to very much nutritional support.

But I needed to feel that I was in motion, doing something, and finding solutions. So I started to research — YouTube and the Internet became my friends as I looked for answers to this rare kind of leukemia. We didn't have access to the chemotherapy drugs yet and, anyway, I wasn't sure how I felt about them. Nutritionally, I decided I needed more detox, even though the month of double pneumonia had already been a detox. Without even trying, I had cut calories drastically, taken out processed food, and mindfully ate unprocessed, simple mono meals, not even mixing food too much. In two weeks I had lost 20 pounds and my blood pressure had dropped to a low of 93/60. I had struggled with the breathing but finally got my oxygen back. My thinking had become clearer, but looking for information on the Internet was still overwhelming. It's not easy to process information when you're highly stressed. A family member from Denmark suggested that I take papaya seeds. I did try that occasionally with honey but not on a regular basis. One friend mentioned the benefits of Chaga mushrooms. Supposedly they are very good for prevention and detoxification, but I didn't have the strength to look it up and would have had to find a Chinese herbal doctor. There were such doctors close to where we lived, but I didn't have the energy to go through the translating process. My friend also mentioned Toco powder, high enzymes, and Insulin Potentiation Therapy — using insulin so that a lower dose of chemotherapy is needed. Regardless of whether the treatments were good or bad, I had never heard of any them and it was difficult to do all the research.

I decided that I needed to detox… my mind, my emotions, and my body. I wanted to give myself the best chance for my immune system to do the job of helping me get healthy. I was going to treat my sickness as a challenge. In my mind, the diet part of the detox would mean taking out processed foods and supplementing with vitamins/herbs considered to be antioxidants.

"One of the first duties of the physician is to educate the masses not to take medicine." William Osler (1849-1919)

Q. Do you think food can help prevent or destroy cancer cells?

Part of the detox: *Eating Whole, Unprocessed Foods*

Hippocrates said, "Let food be thy medicine and medicine be thy food." I see this quote everywhere now and it is so profound! If you search for this quote, there are endless memes, inspiring people to eat whole foods, green foods, fruits, and everything from nature. Another way to say this is that every time you are eating something, you are either feeding disease or fighting disease. I felt this! I wanted to know that everything I put in my body was going to help get rid of cancer or, more importantly, help my body get rid of cancer and find balance again.

When I say this I see little soldiers inside my body. I often tried to brainwash my kids against too much sugar. I told them that gummy bears were made from pig bone and for some time they thought this was disgusting and wouldn't eat any candies made with gelatin. Unfortunately, the attraction of gummy bears was often stronger than my analogy. Another comparison is the idea of "soldier cells" in their body, ready to fight any foreign "enemy" — substances or bad germs. So whenever my kids eat too much sugar, their soldiers get sleepy and can't fight against the bad cells, which will start making them sick. I like the visual component of this analogy. I just knew that I didn't need as much sugar (added or inherent) as I was taking in every day. The American Heart Association recently declared that we don't need more than 9 teaspoons (36 grams) of added sugar for men and 6 teaspoons (24 grams) for women a day. To visualize this, a tablespoon is 4 grams of sugar. So a couple cups of coffee with sugar could easily reach the limit, without even looking at cereals, crackers, salad dressings, pasta sauces, or desserts! Even an organic cereal bar might have 15 grams of sugar. A serving of baby carrots and an ear of corn have 13 grams of sugar. All this means that even without any addition of refined sugar, we will get more than enough carbohydrates from fruits, vegetables, and complex grains. Government health associations around the world are constantly changing their recommendations, but it's not hard to see that added refined sugar is one of the main culprits against health.

I saw a cartoon showing a farmer working behind the "Farmacy." He was handing out a bag of carrots and lettuce and saying, "Take one a day." It's true – an apple a day <u>does</u> keep the doctor away. I took this slogan seriously: I was going to focus on real, unprocessed foods.

I started my detox. I took out refined sugar and starchy grains that might cause inflammation. Instead, I focused on eating fruits and vegetables, lots of raw food, limited slow- cook rice, quinoa, healthier cereal options, and small amounts of protein. I included chia seeds, lemon juice, apple cider vinegar, coconut oil, plant-based protein powder, hemp seeds, walnuts, and almonds into my daily routine. I added several supplements including: 1000 mg Vit C, B6/B12, Calcium/magnesium, Spirulina, Zinc, Selenium, Astralagus, CoQ10, Tumeric, Cinnamon, Milk Thistle, and some papaya seeds. It's not a perfect list, but I felt the supplements would do what I wanted – help give my body the boost it needed in case I wasn't getting enough vitamins from the food. I was looking for antioxidant and liver cleansing support.

I had to be careful with protein, however. I needed it as was anemic from the low red blood cell count, but many health food advocates warned of the toxicity of animal protein. This would mean my body would have to work harder to get rid of those toxins while my system was already stressed. There was lots of research that spoke of cancer feeding and developing in an acidic environment and that trying to dominate my diet with alkaline foods would promote my detox further.

My trainer pointed me in the direction of the Gerson Diet, developed by Max Gerson, a German-born American in the early part of the 20th-century. His daughter, Charlotte Gerson, has inspiring information on several websites. The basis is that diet can control cancer and other chronic conditions. One of the main aspects is the concentrated amount of juicing each day. I wasn't motivated to follow the exact plan but I liked the idea of juicing. I needed the concentrated amount of vitamins, flavonoids and antioxidants to support my detox. I couldn't eat the number of nutrients in one day that the juices would quickly provide. I varied from one to five juices per day, focusing on beet and green vegetable juices. I had an enlarged spleen and if you ask a Chinese medicine practitioner, the spleen is related to blood issues. How to improve the blood? Some health food promoters will talk about beet and cherry juice. Does the fact that both beet and cherry juice are red have something to do with it? I was a bit skeptical but was willing to give it a try. Luckily, I had a nanny who also helped in the house. It is a lot of work to make juices throughout the day. I am not sure I would recommend it to someone who just wants to be healthy or lose a few pounds. Having the whole green vegetable in a smoothie with all the fiber provides many benefits over the juicing, but I needed my vitamins quickly. Juicing was a fast track to boosting my immune system.

Q. Do you ever think about what is happening in your gut?

Part of the detox: *Healing the Gut*

At one point in the detox, I realized that even though I was eating a super healthy diet, I didn't seem to be absorbing all the nutrients and vitamins in my food. I started researching the link between gut health and overall health, and the strength or weakness of the immune system. If the analogy about sugar was little soldiers getting sleepy with fast food and treats, then my gut was like a whole city of citizens. From a philosophical perspective, it's quite amazing how much is happening in the gut; most of us are oblivious to the millions of cells and constant activity inside our gut and bloodstream. If we are the specks in a collection of galaxies, then we are also the whole to the sum of our inner cells and organs. In a recent article, Laura Sanders speaks of how "human and bacterial cells evolved together, like a pair of entwined trees, growing and adapting into a (mostly) harmonious ecosystem."[2]

I never thought about my gut bacteria, and how vital they are. The list of benefits of healthy gut bacteria is extensive. It can:

1) Crowd out pathogens

2) Help your body absorb nutrients

3) Keep the PH balanced

4) Produce digestive enzymes

---

2   Sanders, L. (2016, April 2) Microbes can play games with the mind. *Science News: Magazine of the Society for Science & the Public*, 189 (7), 23.

5) Modulate genes

6) Synthesize hormones

7) Synthesize fat-soluble vitamins

8) Synthesize B-complex vitamins

9) Digest food

10) Train the immune system to distinguish friend from foe and a few more jobs. [3]

With so many important roles, it's no wonder that an imbalance of gut bacteria could lead to symptoms such as bloating, leaky gut, gluten intolerance, eczema, thyroid disorders, weight problems, fatigue, and brain fog. [4]

How could cancer cells develop inside us? From a nature perspective, shouldn't we be designed to heal ourselves and become healthy? Author and leader in functional medicine, Dr. Alejandro Junger, has a great analogy, comparing our gut to a country's homeland security system with many divisions. [5] Our immune system is ready to fight bacteria, viruses, allergic reactions, and cancer cells with a variety of different kinds of cells. He likens cancer cells to terrorist cells in a city gone awry. So if I am providing my system with healthy foods and few pollutants, my gut citizens will be happy and continue doing what they need to do to keep me healthy. But if

---

3   Chutkan, R., *The Microbiome Solution: A Radical New Way to Heal Your Body from the Inside Out* (Penguin Random House: New York, 2015) p. 12.

4   Chutkan, R., *The Microbiome Solution: A Radical New Way to Heal Your Body from the Inside Out* (Penguin Random House: New York, 2015) p. 15.

5   Junger, A., *Clean Gut: The Breakthrough Plan for Eliminating the Root Cause of Disease and Revolutionizing Your Health* (Harper One, 2013) p. 65.

my system is bombarded with stress, toxicity, and unhealthy foods, the cancer cells will become terrorists who think they are doing what's right for the city in protest but are actually causing more harm. Somehow, this analogy was comforting to me. It gave me a way to make peace with my cancer cells. They just didn't know any better and it was my job to help my immunity cells fight them.

There were a lot of different suggested strategies for supporting gut health, including strange self-made videos of people who were ingesting a lot of baking soda concoctions. I was aware of trying to chew my food for a longer time and not to drink water with a meal. I also changed to stronger probiotics. I could only get 50 million counts but would have gone with 100 billion. I already liked the occasional kimchi with my vegetables and added it more often, increasing fermented foods. Other suggestions included: peppermint tea, digestive enzymes, and avoiding cold drinks; for a while, I used wormwood oil, in case there were any parasites I hadn't noticed. It was already a given that I eliminate coffee, black tea, and alcohol from my diet. I was determined to be kind to my digestive system. I think the biggest help for my gut was apple cider vinegar. I had it every morning an hour or so after breakfast. I usually aimed for a third of a cup with a cup of room temperature water. It took some getting used to but I believe it helped. By detoxing my gut, I was getting to the source of my illness that could lead to the spread of new health.

Q. Do you feel your emotional health can affect your body's well being?

Part of the detox: *Attitude*

I always find it interesting that whenever I start getting the sniffles I sometimes get a cold and sometimes I don't. What are the daily micro changes in the cells that lead them toward health or sickness? I suppose if I had the answer I would already be a millionaire but the world of our ever-changing cells has so many contributing factors.

I do believe the power of my mind affects my health. If I believe that there's a bug going around that everyone's catching, then I will most likely get sick. If I believe I might not catch the bug, depending on my own immunity, I might not get sick. I always blame myself when I get sick, wondering what I could have done to prevent it. Emotional wellness is key to health, even though the link between the mind and the body might not be totally understood.

I already said it, but it's worth repeating: having cancer is stressful. When you get this diagnosis it's pretty hard not to constantly think about what's happening in your body. While my blood tests were still showing worsening numbers, I had a fear of the bad cells in my body and that nothing was being done to stop them. A lot of people who get cancer suffer from depression following a diagnosis or ongoing treatment. There is almost a neurosis of fear that the depression is going to make cancer worse. I was staying positive but there was still worry that if I let depression take over, my body wouldn't heal. I also had a fear that if I tried to go against my natural feelings, the asynchrony of my mind would have a worse effect on my health. How to be true to your feelings when you're busy trying to craft what kind of feelings would result in the best health?

Feeling stressed about being stressed was a never-ending (and nonsensical) situation. I remembered getting sick after pulling all-nighters at university and keeping things going until the last paper was handed; then a cold set in. I needed to respect any feelings of fear, anger, and depression that I had and then figure out how to support myself with positivity and affirmation. I had to listen to what my gut was telling me with changing emotions that didn't have a rulebook. It's not difficult to find examples of what stress does to people every day – in hair, skin, weight, and wrinkles. I couldn't afford the effects of stress with my blood count already dominated by cancer.

I also knew that I needed to be motivated. I couldn't give up the fight against cancer. We're always taught in school to never give up, just like "The Little Engine that Could." I was brainwashed with the "I think I can" mentality. My sister said that I was being very brave. My response was "what other choice did I have?" Around me, my children and husband were coping but eagerly waiting for me to get better so that we could get back to our normal lives. They needed me. Some people give up when things go wrong, and others don't. What makes some people more resilient? I am not sure – but I love reading inspirational quotes and getting motivated by others who overcome challenges and rise to greatness. I distinctly remember two posters we had on the wall as children. One was above the hall mirror, where we would sit and do our hair before school. It said, "A smile is a frown upside down." The other was a big wall poster with a picture of the back of a child running with a kite. It read, "Today is the first day of the rest of your life." Perhaps I was brainwashed to stay resilient at an early age.

My Australian friends told me about the amazing affirmations of an American motivational author, Louise Hay. I believed in affirmation but had been lazy to try it in the past. Now, as part of the detox, I searched the Internet for something that rang true to me and that I wouldn't forget to do. I found this: I accept and love myself completely as I am. I put it on the bathroom mirror and promised myself I would read it aloud every morning. There is something powerful about saying something out loud, instead of in your head. It makes things real and you can hear the emotion in your voice. I didn't want a quote specifically about fighting cancer. I needed something that allowed me to love myself regardless of illness, so I would avoid feelings of guilt, shame, or regret. The cancer was in my blood and part of who I was at the time. In order to get well, I had to listen to the little voice inside that told me to keep up a good attitude.

Q. Do you ever feel like you just need a rest to get better when you're sick?

Part of the detox: Rest

There was a time when I didn't really respect the need for sleep. Obviously, this was before I had children. Whether it was university deadlines, Masters presentations, or teaching projects, there were many times when sleep was put on hold because I wanted to make a deadline or do my best job. I figured I could catch up on what I needed on my days off. If it was only a few hours, this worked, but over time the side effects were more noticeable. When the kids were babies, I craved sleep and found it hard to think, as most moms could attest to. With cancer, I believed that my body needed the rest. It was during sleep that the magic happened. Cells went to work... processing, healing, and regenerating. I was already close to fainting most of the time; I knew I didn't want to overtire my compromised immune system.

It's likely that all the resting I did was really a form of subconscious meditation or prayer. Half the time, I wasn't sleeping but I wasn't thinking about anything either; often just focused on willing my fever to come down, willing the shakes to stop, or counting my breathing to relax. Without the mind racing, my body had the focus and energy to respond to the daily challenges. I knew that concentrating my mind would help me make decisions, lessen any anxiety, boost my immune system, and maybe even improve my brain function!

Another kind of rest is digestive rest. A lot of people talk about fasting during detox but there is also research on intermittent fasting — giving the body a break from all the meals and constant digesting. We all eat less when we're sick and patients are advised to take fluids and rest. When I look at my kids, they are having a daily intermittent fast. They eat dinner at 6 pm and don't eat again until 8 am. That's a 14-hour break from eating and digesting. Why shouldn't I do the same? I knew I didn't need the late evening snack, giving me a restless sleep or a morning stomachache. Whilst trusting my body to heal itself, the fourth aspect of my detox was rest.

My Facebook post on April 2014:

1000 mg vit c, milk thistle, spirulina, evening primrose oil, coconut oil, flax seeds, brewer's yeast, calcium/magnesium, B6/12, omega 3, selenium, positive affirmation, cider vinegar, 4 strain probiotics, green juices

& red juices, chia seed cereal, green tea, raw veggies &
fruit, low amount of starchy carbs, iron… am I missing
anything for getting healthy?

The most intense part of this diet — without sugar, processed foods or acidic foods — lasted for four weeks. It was
a full-time job. A typical day started with lemons and hot
water. I always had water with me and aimed for three liters a
day. Breakfast might be eggs and avocado or chia seeds soaked
in almond milk. I should have made my own almond milk
but the task never made it to the top of the list. It took me a
long time to get showered and dressed since I had to rest after
each step so I wouldn't faint. I practiced speaking my daily
affirmation and then I would work on breathing and mindfulness. I would have vitamins later in the morning so as not
to feel nauseous but I often fell asleep for an hour. I would
work on Hairy Cell Leukemia research on the Internet or
respond to messages on email and Facebook. I would check
my oxygen level, my temperature, and my blood pressure
throughout the day. I would have some vegetables for lunch,
keeping things raw and adding nuts or seeds. After lunch, I
would work on visualization or reading or listen to music and
wait for my helper to come to make some juices. I needed to
rest after lunch to save up energy for my kids after school. I
couldn't leave the chair or bed too long without feeling faint,
so there wasn't too much action. Dinner was vegetables and
quinoa or a bit of rice or protein.

Looking back, the diet wasn't complicated, but putting
all the parts together made it into a complete detox.

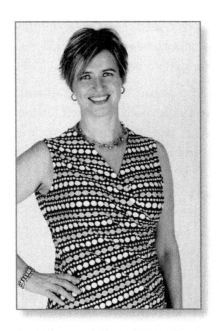

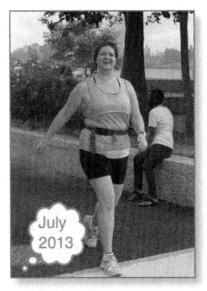

Chapter 4.
How can I get my drugs?

One of the reasons I had so much time to focus on a detox to boost my immune system was that the chemotherapy drugs, which were the regular protocol for Hairy Cell Leukemia, were not available in Macau. Usually, doctors rush patients into a protocol without much time to weigh the pros and cons of chemotherapy. Since I was at a University Hospital and the consulting doctor was mainly a researcher, he spent time discussing the medical options with me. Maybe he also realized that I needed to feel in control of the discussion, and sent me home with photocopies of some of the studies of the protocol. However, as I mentioned previously, Hairy Cell Leukemia is relatively rare since so few people have it and, therefore, few studies had been done into this disease. As far as I could decipher the educational and scientific jargon, one study from Japan looked like solid research but it was conducted with fewer than 100 participants! Whatever limited research I read reassured me of the positive results of chemotherapy in treating HCL, but also gave me some room for flexibility in the protocol.

My doctor and Paddy were trying hard to get access to the chemotherapy drugs, but I was happy that they weren't readily available in Macau so I had time to think about my action plan. The word "chemotherapy" did not evoke positive thoughts in me. There are so many sites on the Internet that not only promote alternate therapies for cancer but also actively oppose chemotherapy. The main argument, of course, is that chemotherapy drugs not only kill bad cells but also good cells and weaken the immune system at the same time. It is not hard to believe that a patient who appears sick during cancer treatment looks that way from the effects of the chemo, rather than cancer itself.

Q. Do you know someone who has debated using traditional chemotherapy or alternative treatments?

As a patient, I felt stuck in the middle. On one hand, it is hard to wade through the propaganda from the world of alternative health; on the other, it is difficult to read scientific journals when your brain is a bit foggy from sickness. Why can't there be a happy Venn diagram intersection of alternative and current western medicine with the patient in the middle? It would be like a huge health hug. When I lived in Taiwan, I appreciated the holistic perspective of Chinese medicine doctors, who looked at a wide spectrum of symptoms to make a diagnosis. In the North American world of health advocates, Dr. Mark Hyman often talks about the value of functional medicine –looking at the underlying cause of disease, rather than just treating symptoms. I appreciate doctors who want to engage me towards optimal health, believing in the body's ability to regulate and get rid of disease.

There are several health advocates who have found health without chemotherapy. One example is Kris Carr - a brave woman who maintains her health after being diagnosed with multiple tumors that were not treatable with chemotherapy. She has been living and thriving with eHAE (Epithelioid haemangioendothelioma) for more than a decade, and focuses on plant-based recipes and juicing. Another advocate of finding health without chemotherapy is Chris Wark who, at 26, was diagnosed with Stage 3 colon cancer that had spread to the lymph nodes. He agreed to surgery but then refused chemotherapy against the advice of his doctors, and went on to become healthy through alternative lifestyle and nutritional routines.

However, I couldn't mention any of these people to my consulting oncologist. He was a smart researcher, but alternate practices were not on his radar. He was focused on mainstream medicine and its results. Holland (2001) states that 85% of people in the U.S.A. resort to conventional cancer treatments, while at the same time trying to add on complementary treatments to get the best of both worlds.[6] That was my case as well. I didn't have the energy to argue with my husband and I was too scared to say no to chemotherapy completely, but I had to look at other ways to get healthy again.

Cladribine (2-chlorodeoxyadenosine) under the Trade name, Leustatin®, was the medication my doctor was looking for. Since there are very few people requesting this drug, it wasn't readily available in Macau. As we couldn't get the chemotherapy drugs right away, the doctor suggested another medication, Rituximab (under the trade name, Rituxan®),

---

6   Holland, J. C. & S. Lewis, *The Human Side of Cancer: Living with Hope, Coping with Uncertainty* (Quill: New York, 2000) p. 181.

also used for HCL. The usual protocol was to offer this drug to patients who didn't respond to the standard chemotherapy drugs or to those who weren't strong enough to handle Cladribine. The majority of the patients with HCL were middle-aged to senior men with possibly an already weaker immune system. I didn't really understand what a monoclonal antibody drug was, how it worked, or what the side effects were but it seemed commonly used and how could I say no to the doctor? I didn't have any other alternatives. I could say it was our decision, but essentially it was the doctor's: he offered a solution where a non-standard protocol of Rituximab first would bring up my red cell counts in the short term, preparing my immune system in the long term to be able to handle the chemotherapy when we could access it. I didn't know what the plan was going to be to get the Cladribine. The doctor assured us that he would take care of it.

Rituximab is a monoclonal antibody used in cancer treatment and other illnesses, but not a chemotherapy drug. Now I understand that it is a type of immunotherapy treatment, aiming to boost one's own immune system. Another type of immunotherapy treatment is the development of cancer vaccines. Although not without side effects, I kind of like the idea of helping the immune system, instead of killing off both good and bad cells.

Rituximab works by binding to the CD20 protein found on B cells, and killing off B cells (including healthy and cancerous cells), thus giving the body an opportunity to develop new cells from the lymphoid stem cells. It's on the World Heath Organization's list of Essential Medicines deemed necessary in a basic health system. But recently, it has been reclassified as a specialty drug and hospitals will need to pay more to get it. I qualified for free health care at the government hospital but the staff there didn't have experience with this kind of cancer or the ability to acquire the drugs we had decided on for protocol. Rituximab is easy to access but very expensive — something like 4000 USD for each session — so I can imagine why it's not offered much in the government-sponsored Canadian medical system. I was in shock to realize the costs of medicine. The plan was to have one session a week, for four weeks. I was so grateful for my husband's foresight to get private medical insurance that we could access to reclaim most of our expenses. It was a lot of money to shell out for something that was actually like a poison.

I was just getting better from double pneumonia, but had already had a couple of blood transfusions. They gave me the boosts I needed to keep from fainting and get me out of the bed or a chair, even it was just to get showered and get to my doctor appointments. I wasn't really sure what I was saying yes to. The Rituximab drug treatments were only once a week for a month and gave me more time to think about my position on the chemotherapy. I didn't realize the full effects of what I was going to put into my body! Since I was at a training hospital, the nurses were not familiar with the drug. The first session was going to take several hours, as the doctor didn't know how I would react to the drug. I was relieved when he said he would be monitoring me for side effects. He sat there for four hours, watching me. I was happy that he could spend time taking care of me, but it most likely also reflected the serious reactivity of the drug. He gave me a paper from the bottle that explained the possible side effects but the writing was very small and the list was so long; I didn't want to get anxious by reading it all. I knew that my blood pressure and heart rate were already rising.

When the intravenous drip started, it was very bizarre to feel the drug going through my veins. It was on the verge of painful as if I was being poisoned. As soon as I thought that, I had to push this idea out of my head. How could I think that something poisonous would help me? I had to visualize that this drug was helping me and imagine new health. I started a fever, which was easy enough to counteract. But after half an hour, I began shaking. I didn't think much of it until I shook so much that my teeth were chattering uncontrollably. Without thinking, I put my knuckles in my mouth to stop from biting my tongue. It was almost unbearable —as if I had spent a night in the snow and every part of my body was now shivering. I couldn't lay still. The doctor gave me something to stop the shaking. I was forever grateful since even 15 minutes of this intense shaking felt so long. Finally, whatever I had been given to counteract side effects led me into a warm fuzzy daze.

The "what to expect" info for Rituxan® warns that the first infusion would last between four and six hours and that the patient should bring along a book or some music to pass the time. But there was no way I could have read, as all my energy went into surviving the side effects! Most of the side effects from immunotherapy treatment are basically severe allergic reactions but several include serious, life-threatening infections. I am glad I didn't read the fine print, or I might have chickened out. The next time around, I was given a whole series of medicine before the session started, to counteract the side effects of the previous week. I was grateful at the time but didn't realize that I was probably given some steroids as well, and it would take months to undo their effects.

After each session, I would still be extremely dozy. Later in the evenings, all my bones would hurt. It was as if the drug was still moving through my body. Sitting on the sofa, I would often start shaking again. I couldn't sit still yet could barely walk, and would ask my husband to hold me, willing the shaking to stop so that I could go to sleep. I was grateful this treatment was only once a week; on the other days, I'd concentrate on willing the side effects to go away so I would be ready for the next session.

Q. Why is one's person's illness not a good enough reason to order drugs?

I asked my doctor a couple of times how he was going to get the chemotherapy drug that we had planned to use next. He didn't have a straight answer yet. I continued with my detox, nutritional and lifestyle research, and getting through the weekly side effects of the Rituximab. I was focusing on alternative therapies but in the back of my mind, I was still a bit stressed about not having the chemotherapy drug available. I needed to have a plan to feel in control. My doctor had asked the local pharmaceutical company to order in the Cladribine. He was a consulting doctor and not a resident of the country so his request might have had less authority. I was a resident of Macau but an expatriate. I wondered if being an outsider limited my power as well. The pharmaceutical company denied the request for the drug, stating that it wasn't worth the cost to bring it in for one person. Whether I was in North America, Europe or Southeast Asia, I was used to being able to get what I needed when I needed it. Although sometimes costs were higher, the options were always there. Now I felt like a peon on the outside of a big business. I couldn't just snap my fingers and have my request granted. I was shocked by the amount of power a pharmaceutical company had on my health – that they could decide if one person's health was a viable expenditure or not! But my doctor did not give up. He was speaking at a conference and mingled with other physicians, asking for their help. He found out that Taiwan had enough Cladribine for two patients, and one doctor he'd never met before agreed to ask the hospital she worked at for help. The hospital said no, pointing to the fact that I wasn't a resident of Taiwan. She went to her previous workplace, a teaching hospital, which said yes; providing that I had the drug administered in their hospital. I didn't want to stay in Taiwan to have the chemo, but I knew there would be room to negotiate. When I lived in Taiwan and welcomed new expat teachers to the school, I always had two bits of advice for them: 1) Whenever you think you know what's going on, you don't... and 2) Everything always works out – just not always in the most direct way.

By this time, I had gone through the weeks of double pneumonia and another four weeks of nutritional detox, plus the four sessions of Rituximab. I had had a couple of blood transfusions but after the Rituximab, my red cell count was going up a bit. Things were happening according to plan. My doctor didn't think the Rituximab would work in the long term, but that it would work in the few weeks I needed to be ready for chemotherapy. The next step would be up to me. I had to be the negotiator and get my drugs. It wouldn't be a good idea for my husband to go on his own or travel with me, as we didn't want to gang up on the doctors; besides, I needed him home to watch the kids. "Saving face" in Taiwan was a big consideration when negotiating. I decided I would stay overnight and come back the next day. I was grateful that my doctor had found the Cladribine, but part of me resented having to make the trip on my own, having to go to another country just to negotiate for my own drugs! On one hand, I was ready to be strong – to do what was needed. But on the other, I was thinking, "I have cancer. Please, someone take care of me. I don't want to be strong." These thoughts triggered deep issues. I did want to be strong and practiced leadership skills to gain confidence. I am the oldest child. I like having control. I am tall with Scandinavian and German heritage. There isn't anything slight about me. But I am also sensitive and need time to recharge my energy after being around lots of people. Emotions are at the forefront of all my exchanges with others. The thought of the trip ahead made me sigh. Why did I have to be the strong fighter again?

Q. When you are sick, do you take charge of your health routine or have others take care of you, or both?

It wasn't too long a trip but I took everything slowly. Walking through customs, finding a train, looking at maps, finding a taxi – everything took time, as well as physical and mental energy. I was constantly breathing hard and gauging when I could next sit down. When I got to the hospital, I was so grateful for the Taiwanese doctor who had arranged everything for my visit. She was there as a total stranger, yet she and her assistant volunteered several hours of their day to help me. I had experienced the gentleness of the Taiwanese culture when I lived there before, but I was still overwhelmed by the kindness of strangers whilst I was feeling so vulnerable as a patient. Trying to negotiate the logistics and map of a hospital would have been a struggle on my own, not being able to read the signs. I tried my best to keep track of what was happening. There were papers to be filled, fees to pay, blood tests to be taken, and lines to wait in. The idea was that the doctor helping me (let's call her Ms. Lee) would introduce me to the oncologist, her previous teacher and mentor (let's call him Mr. Wu). We waited outside Mr. Wu's office, while I tried to make small talk with Ms. Lee. I started realizing that my red cell count must have been very low because even though I was trying to be sociable, Ms. Lee kept asking if I was okay. I was used to walking around while feeling faint, but I probably didn't look too well from everyone else's perspective. I was paying attention to the others waiting in the hallway and noticed some hospital workers talking to patients. Ms. Lee told me that these women were not only volunteers; they were previous patients themselves, cancer survivors who could both relate to and encourage the other patients. As survivors, these women felt obliged to contribute to the hospital and volunteer their time. I was amazed at their generosity and service to other patients. I was focused on being patient as a patient! It was finally our turn, and the negotiation could start. Mr. Wu could speak English, but there was still a bit of a communication barrier and I chose my words carefully. He looked at my history and listened to my story. He agreed that I should have the Cladribine, but stated that I needed to have repeat courses for a couple of months and had to stay in the hospital following the chemotherapy to recover when my numbers would initially drop. Inside my head, I started to panic a bit. I didn't want a repeat course of chemo and I certainly didn't want to recover in the Taiwan hospital; but most of all, I didn't want to have the chemo in Taiwan at all. I started to explain that my doctor had decided on a protocol of only one week of treatment and that I was worried to leave my kids alone for too long. As a mother of young kids, I needed to get back to them as soon as possible. I suggested that if I stayed in Taiwan to take 5 days of treatment, I could fly back to Macau straight away before any of my numbers dropped or I got sick from the chemotherapy. I tried to call my doctor in Macau, but he wasn't picking up his cell phone. I was on my own to figure this out. Ms. Lee and Mr. Wu spoke in Mandarin for a bit and all of a sudden he changed his mind. I think he realized that my protocol was so different from what his hospital normally followed, that he didn't want to get involved with something complicated. He agreed that I could take the Cladribine back to Macau with me but that he had to order it from the pharmacy and I would have to come back a week later to pick it up. I happily agreed, not complaining about another airplane flight I would have to take in a week.

After a few hours, it started to rain. It was also rush hour everyone so was trying to get home. Again, I saw the doctors' generosity when Ms. Lee's assistant volunteered to walk me the two blocks in the rain to the hotel and carried my suitcase. When I got to the hotel, I called Paddy to tell him the good news and then focused on getting some food and being able to relax for the rest of the evening. I didn't have to walk far to shops underground by the metro station to find what I needed.

Facebook: "Forgot how much I love Taiwan! Smiling shopkeepers and friendly strangers; almonds & dried fish much better than Pringles; bok choy & rice for fast food, served faster than McDonald's; and flexible doctors!" (May 1)

One week later, I flew to Taiwan to get the Cladribine. I planned a day trip, so I could get everything over with, but I knew it would be a long day. I was grateful for the support of friends around me, as one of my workout friends drove me to the airport. I didn't want to look sick to cause attention while traveling, and started off the day in a smart casual outfit, putting out my best energy but struggled to get in and out of the car when my friend picked me up. She had just come from a workout and was bustling around doing errands. I was quick to notice the sharp contrast in our energies, as I knew all I had done that morning was get ready for the trip. This trip felt harder than the previous one. I was nervous to eat anything so as not to have a stomach upset but also nervous to not eat as I needed the energy. Even sitting down for two hours on the plane and then on the train into town was difficult. I was on my own this time and tried to remember how to find my way around the hospital, without having to ask too many people for help. Another difference this time was that I was carrying a wallet of cash – about $5000 USD in Taiwanese bills, to pay for my drugs! I met Mr. Wu again, thanked him profusely before he could change his mind, paid him, got the drug, and headed back to the airport. By the time I was waiting for the airplane I was exhausted. I had stressed a bit going through customs, as I didn't know how they would react to me bringing Cladribine out of the country. I was carrying 10 individual liquid vials with a paper signed by the hospital, giving me permission to have the drug. Individuals didn't normally carry drugs like this on their own, so I didn't know what the reaction would be. I shouldn't have worried; the customs officer hardly glanced when I held up the bag I was carrying! I went to rest in the waiting area and kept on my face mask and sunglasses to stay protected. My selfie that day looked like an odd cross between strong fighter and vulnerable patient.

> Facebook: "Step 5 completed and bringing chemo drugs back to Macau. Feel like crap -but seem to be blending in with the locals. I am giving myself a pat on the back and God bless Taiwan!" (May 8)

The next day I spent most of the time on the sofa (while the kids played around me), trying to gain my strength back to get ready for the chemotherapy on Monday morning.

> Facebook: "5:30am wake up on a rainy day = iPad surfing, looking at rocks, Lego, breakfast, looking through old toy box, dancing, indoor football, jobs, snack, trampoline, Lego, jungle animals, puppies, helping Daddy in the garage, clean up, lunch, book reading, playing with stuffed animals, some napping, some movie, snack, road making craft, colouring & drawing, car play, marble tower and finally dinner time while mommy monitored fairly immobile from the sofa" (May 10)

That evening, I was in more pain than I could ever imagine – detoxing a month of chia seeds? Exposed hemorrhoids and open sores and trying not to faint in the shower. I didn't put that on Facebook.

Chapter 5.
What's it like to have chemo?

The kids were fine but I felt bad to be away from them on my trip to Taiwan. Now it was the weekend and it was raining and we were all in the apartment, competing for space. My husband was on the computer a lot; I could barely move from the sofa in pain from the newly acquired hemorrhoids and the energetic twins wanted to play throughout the day. They managed fine. Life went on, regardless of whether or not I was sick. One day my friend took the twins for the afternoon. Despite my endless "mom guilt," the children now hardly remember me being sick but they do remember having an afternoon in town going bowling with their friend and his family.

Years ago my grandfather was diagnosed with lung cancer. He'd already had heart attacks and was a faithful smoker of Camel cigarettes. He never talked about his diagnosis. One afternoon, as a precocious teenager, I pushed my grandfather to talk about his feelings about cancer, believing that keeping all the emotions bottled up inside was doing more harm. He remained stubborn, yet got upset that I was getting upset. There was never a question of chemotherapy or drug treatment. He just wanted to keep living the way he had been living. I guess he knew that the treatment would not have helped him at such a late stage. Would other treatments have helped? Maybe they would have bought him more time. But he wanted to ignore the diagnosis – maybe it was too hard to accept the finality of what was going to happen.

So did I believe the chemotherapy was going to help? What was my mindset before starting the week of treatments? I didn't want to take the perspective of fighting cancer because having leukemia meant that the cancer was already in my blood cells. This was not just one tumor —an enemy invader – that I could fight against. Therefore, I didn't want to think of the chemotherapy attacking cancer. It didn't feel right. If I only thought of controlling cancer, this implied having to fight something against myself. How could I fight against myself? I think this would create a dichotomy in the body and cause more stress and anxiety. When I hear the word "control," I get a negative reaction. I think of going against the flow and struggling with something. But I still wanted to be an active participant in my health. I didn't want to be passive. I needed to figure out how chemotherapy was going to work for me. I think my husband would have freaked out if I had refused chemo. It was scary to say no, though part of me wanted to.

I had a lot of slogans in my head from people who are sure that chemotherapy kills more than it helps; that I was putting poison into your body; and that chemo was western medicine's only hope in an area they were still floundering to understand. There are many reports that chemotherapy feeds the cancer business wheel, giving false hope and continued funds to big pharma corporations. As I had already discovered when trying to access my medications, the drug companies did not always have the needs of individual patients in mind. While trying to research the effectiveness of the Cladribine, I stumbled upon numerous warning letters issued by Regulatory Review Officers of the Drug Marketing, Advertising & Communications Division of the FDA and directed to various pharmaceutical companies that were not accurate in their representation of the negative effects of the drugs they were selling. There are many anti-chemotherapy websites that promote alternative naturopathic drugs. Was chemotherapy being ineffective by not killing the sick cells but poisoning healthy ones instead? One of the warnings about Cladribine is that it has clastogenic effects. This means that it can cause DNA damage by deleting, adding, or rearranging chromosomes. I did not know this before I received the drug. This seems dramatic to me but would it have influenced my decision to take or not take the drug if I had read this information prior to treatment? I really don't know. It might have given me a reason beyond my own instinctive fear to use as an excuse not to take Cladribine.

In contrast, there are reports of chemotherapy being very effective in treating (and even curing) leukemia. I realize I am diving into murky waters here. The contradictory studies are so numerous. The passion that each doctor has for opposing points of view is a bit disconcerting to a patient. Even in my current healthy state, I struggle to find the truth that helps patients decide what treatment to choose (or not choose). One of the reasons it's hard to find credible answers is that it's more than just looking for a cure for Cancer with a capital C. Cancer is not really one thing – this term encompasses dozens of diseases with multiple combinations in cell growth irregularities. There are five main categories of cancer, depending on what type of cell cancer starts from:

1) Carcinomas; 2) Sarcomas; 3) Leukemias; 4) Lymphomas
and myeloma (lymphatic system cancers); and 5) Brain and
spinal cord cancers. Each category has several sub-types and
numerous drug options.

Q. What is your definition of cancer treatment?

Treatments for cancer are even more varied. Years ago,
the choices included surgery, radiation, and chemotherapy.
None of these was a great option and the room always went
quiet when someone talked about their diagnosis. Nowadays, trying to research options for treatment is so confusing.
There are more and more possibilities that are both comforting and overwhelming, including immunotherapy (stimulat-
ing one's own immune system to work harder and smarter
to attack cancer cells) and integrative oncology (combining
drugs with both complementary and alternative treatments).
And there are plenty of chemotherapy drugs used for different stages and different kinds of cancer. Another option is
targeted therapy, which includes the first drug treatment I
had, Rituximab. This particular therapy sounds promising as
drugs are developed to biologically target cancer cells without disturbing the healthy cells, but there are several categories of targeted therapy and numerous drug choices again. It
appears that some medications are more effective with some
cancers than others. I guess the research is ever changing,
but I wish there was a cheat sheet matrix available. I see a
patient sitting down with the doctor and starting the conversation with the type of cancer that needs to be treated. Then
the doctor can say, "Well this is the drug we usually use for
your kind of cancer and it's 80% effective," or "Sorry, it's only
30% effective." Would that clear and straightforward information help the patient or would he or she just say, "Give

me the drugs," not wanting to risk losing a chance that the medication would help? I guess it depends on the individual patient, but I craved information that would help me make choices about treatment.

Q. Do you think some types of chemotherapy are more effective with some types of cancer?

I decided to choose some fight songs because I was fighting to create a positive focus to accept the chemo without my immune system dropping too much. Months later, I was in Starbucks and it was Fight Cancer Month with a donation box and a symbol of daffodils. It gave me the image of an army of patients rallying around the cancer enemy, ready to strike with whatever weapons their imagination could gather. It was a bit comical to me and possibly not realistic. A few days later at home, I heard a knock at the door and I was greeted by two young people, asking for cancer society donations, unaware that I was a cancer survivor myself. Such a mix of emotions struck me. I knew these youngsters were enthusiastic and energetic, and I appreciated their sincerity, trying to do good in the world. But I also felt triggered. Part of me wanted to shock them a bit by throwing at them some tidbits of suffering to question if the cancer society was really there to help me? Another part of me wanted to hear facts. The poor kids weren't ready for my questions. But how could I be reassured that money I gave was going to prevent me from getting leukemia again? I had flashbacks of the pharmaceutical company in Macau not wanting to buy drugs for me. I had some research of the complicated and tainted process by which drug companies obtain patents for new drugs. And I had a feeling that the machinery of cancer foundations needed to be fed. What would happen if we finally had a cure for cancer and no foundations were needed? There would be a lot of people out of work. It's not that I didn't want to be supported and contribute where it would be helpful – but I needed to do more research on my own. The pair left my house — apologetically? Sympathetically? —without a donation.

A week of chemo on Facebook:

May 12 – Day 1

Day one of chemo? No problem - have already had worse things. Thanks mom for letting us listen to Helen Reddy when I was only about ten. The lyrics are still in my head! Good fighting song for Day one! (Listening to "I am Woman" by Helen Reddy, 1975)

May 13 – Day 2

Day two chemo – no problem – Fighting song for the day by Alanis! (Listening to "Crazy" by Alanis Morissette)

May 14 – Day 3

Day 3 chemo + blood transfusion for a bit more gas in the tank - no problem. Fighting song for the day - "Brave" - cheesy video makes me smile (Listening to "Brave," by Sara Bareilles)

May 15 – Day 4

Day 4 chemo – no problem – body's a bit dozy but there's a party in my head (Listening to "Beautiful Life," by Ace of Base)

May 16 – Day 5

Day 5 chemo – Done! I'm not so tough but was brain-washed at an early age – A prime example is this video: "Keep on Moving," by The Brady Bunch

I've always said to my friends that the problem with reality was the lack of background music. I needed music so that I could dictate the atmosphere of what was happening in my life just like a soundtrack to a movie. Having a song focus every day was a way to release emotions that had no words. I had a playlist on my iPod for every chemo session. Why did I do these Facebook posts? Was it my way to keep people involved? Was I trying to motivate myself? Did I need the online cheers from the sidelines to keep my momentum going? I guess it was similar to the time I spent on bed rest during pregnancy. I needed to feel connected but I didn't want people to see me suffering. I wanted to believe in the power of positivity so I was going to bring everyone else along on the sunshine train. There's no way I was going to post anything negative during my week of chemo. The reality? I was suffering so much from my hemorrhoid sores that it took me about two hours to get ready in the morning and I could barely cope with having to sit for the car ride to the hospital. From this perspective, the actual chemo treatment was the least of my worries.

A friend came to visit me one morning in the hospital during the chemo session. It was such a kind gesture and I didn't expect it. I was touched to see her but wasn't feeling great. My automatic reaction was to put on a brave face and smile for the camera. This was evidence of someone having chemo and looking well. I was not going to look like one of the sick people from the stereotypes in my head.

Q. When you think of chemotherapy, what stereotypes come to your mind?

As I previously mentioned, the chemotherapy drug prescribed for Hairy Cell Leukemia is Cladribine. It is a purine analog medication, and although originally developed only for Hairy Cell Leukemia, it is now also used for other blood cancers. This kind of chemotherapy drug works by stopping or slowing down the growth of cancer cells, but it can also harm healthy cells that divide quickly, which suppresses the immune system. Even when the drug was developed in the 1980s, the pharmaceutical companies were not that interested because it was an orphan drug, meaning that it wasn't applicable to any other diseases.

In the science world, chemotherapy medications consist of drugs that kill cancer cells when the cells are dividing and others that kill cells when the cells are at rest. This explains the cycling of chemotherapy treatment. But chemo drugs can't tell the difference between cancer cells and normal cells. So even if normal cells that have been killed off by mistake grow back healthy, there are side effects with other rapidly dividing cells. This explains hair loss, diarrhea, and nausea. I didn't lose my hair, though it seemed to be falling out and growing back at the same time. Although newer drugs have less side effects than when chemotherapy was first developed, each patient reacts differently. I had had eight weeks of diarrhea. I thought it was a result of my extreme detox to raw foods and more vegetables. This was probably also a side effect of so many antibiotics stripping away any natural bacteria in my gut, but I wish the doctor had explained to me the side effects of the chemo medications, as well as the side effects of the drugs given to counteract side effects.

It was great that my doctor helped devise a treatment plan, but his focus was research and drugs, and he was not really familiar with nutrition. During one follow-up appointment, he thought things were going well and I stopped him by complaining about diarrhea and hemorrhoid issues. Since I was having trouble gaining weight, he suggested that I have chocolate and ice cream. My instinct told me this was a bad idea but I was willing to try anything. As you might have guessed, chocolate and ice cream did not agree with my already compromised digestive system. But when I complained again, he was quick to point me towards a nutritionist. Even though there were some language barriers, I was grateful for any support as I felt I had lost track of what my digestion needed. It appeared that the combination of so many weeks of antibiotics had disrupted my digestive tract to the point of robbing my gut of all-important bacteria, along with the bad bacteria. I regained my focus and started thinking of healing my gut bacteria first. The World Cancer Declaration of 2013 stated that one of its targets would be "improving education and training of healthcare professional" (canceratlas.cancer.org). This would be great. Doctors have to do so much training in the types of cancer treatments but receive very little training in nutrition. This probably stems from the history of allopathic medicine in North America and the gradual phasing out of homeopathic doctors from the mainstream, but it is so unbalanced for the patient.

Q. Where do you get your nutritional support information?

During the chemotherapy treatment, there was no doubt that I was sick with cancer. Two weeks into the diagnosis I had lost 20 pounds and my blood pressure was only 93/60. But I still had some pounds to drop and, before my diagnosis, I was still working on losing weight. I had also done the month of detox before the chemo. In a weird way, I was probably healthier than a lot of people, even though I was battling cancer. My skin was better than it had been in months, my eyes were glowing more, and all my clothes were hanging loose. A few weeks before the chemo I wanted to pick up my kids from school. I had just had a blood transfusion the day before and maybe it gave me a boost of energy that lasted a few days. (A blood transfusion was always like getting some more gas in the tank!) I was wearing a dress I hadn't worn in ages and summer sandals for the tropical heat. "You look so good," one of the moms commented. Normally, I would be so excited with this ego-boosting compliment. But she had no idea I lost so much weight because I had been sick - the irony was thick because I had been trying my whole adult life to slim down. She also didn't know how happy I was to overcome my weakness and be able to walk from the car park to the school. There were other things she wasn't aware of either: how much I was sweating because I was so out of shape from all the time spent lying in bed, or how long it took me to shower and dress because of the unbearably painful hemorrhoids. My mind was thinking, "Don't you know I have cancer?" But all I said was "Thank you."

One of the problems with chemotherapy is that all the focus is on the tumor instead of the patient. People look for the outside side effects of what they think chemotherapy will present and if they see someone looking good, they will think, great, she's fine… I don't have to worry. Chemotherapy treatment is a medical option, but I was struggling to be my own advocate. I wanted to look good, but I needed support as well.

It struck home to read the words of author Greg Anderson: "Cancer is not just about the tumor."[7]

One of my sisters reached out to me during the chemo treatment, saying how brave she thought I was. The thing was... I didn't think I was deciding to be brave; I had a husband and two young children. I was doing what I needed to do because there wasn't any other choice. How could I give up on finding health, knowing I would be leaving my family behind? This is what mothers do... whatever needs to be done. During my journey and whenever I needed to work through feelings, I would often sit down to write...

Move
Move until it hurts
Move because it feels good
Move until the tears start
Move until you feel everything
Move until you feel numb
Move because you care
Move because you don't care
Move because there's no other choice

After five days of treatment, it took the rest of the month to start recovery. I thought that maybe I could go back to exercise in a couple of weeks. I didn't like seeing all my muscle disappearing. The problem was that the drugs for leukemia lower blood counts, which means waiting after treatment for blood counts to go back to normal. Subsequently, part of the recovery is the ever-present possibility of getting sick or catching an infection because of the treatment - not cancer! The month of May passed and I was still recovering and also

---

7   Anderson, G. *Cancer: 50 Essential Things to Do* (Plume: New York, 2013) p.10.

trying to improve my digestion. I felt like time was running out. We had booked a family trip to Wales in July. I could see my husband getting tired. He had stopped smoking; taken on more responsibilities with the kids; kept on working; and taken care of me for four months. Of course, he wanted to help me get better, but the stress was taking a toll on him. After he got a psoriasis breakout and a chest infection, I realized that my time as a patient was up. I needed to be a mom and wife again. I didn't want to be the martyr… I wanted to find a balance… but life was calling me.

So off we went to summer holidays in Wales with a busy schedule of visiting family. On one of the few days when I checked my email, there was a surprise note from my doctor:

Dear Gina,

I have performed molecular testing on your samples and did not find any trace of the disease. Will be away 1-4 Aug. Back to work on 5/Aug

Gregory

This message was so off the cuff, almost like an office memo. I was looking for the exclamation marks – You don't have cancer anymore!!! The doctor's nonchalant attitude was prompted by his confidence that the chemotherapy drug would work. I was happy with the news, yet felt odd to read it by email and a bit annoyed at what I interpreted as smugness from the doctor. I don't think it was just the chemotherapy; everything else I had done: affirmations, detox diet, visiting energy healers, rest, and meditation had contributed equally. Getting healthy was life changing, involving more than taking a few drugs and checking it off the list.

How much did the chemotherapy and targeted therapy treatment contribute to my recovery to health? It's hard to know. My immune system had detoxed enough to be ready to receive the chemo so that my body could kick-start a new recovery of building cells. You have to have a minimum of health to handle chemo. My whole lifestyle was altered. My mindset was changed. Everything I did was steering my cells in a new direction… as if you come to a fork in the road and start veering slightly to the left. At first, the change doesn't seem apparent, but after a few months, you've arrived at a completely different destination!

Chapter 6.
Why did I get sick?

It's always the first question in people's minds when something bad happens – especially when someone gets sick. Why did this happen to me?

Whenever I get a cold or a sore throat, I automatically search inwards, asking myself, "What did I do or not do to cause this? Am I stressed? Did I eat something I am sensitive to? What affected my immune system?" I guess some people don't do this kind of introspection. They say, "Oh, yes, I hear it's going around," as a sympathetic response to someone complaining about a recent virus. Last fall, both of my kids had colds. We were in Macau and I was on the phone with my mom in Canada. She replied with empathy, "Oh yes, everyone here has the same thing." You mean this virus was jumping on airplanes and spreading to different continents? Although the spread of infectious diseases often leads to global outbreaks, I just can't accept when people say, "It's going around," as an excuse for my own sore throats, coughs, and sneezes.

Q. Who or what do you blame when you get sick?

Answering the question "why me?" takes on a different magnitude with cancer than with common cold. It certainly blindsided me for a bit when I heard the possible diagnosis of Hairy Cell Leukemia. I realized I was sick but having someone diagnose you with cancer is shocking, to say the least! My first reaction was, "They must be wrong. This is not supposed to happen to me. It doesn't make sense." My second reaction: "What did I do to bring this on? Why has this happened?"

Back in high school, I was constantly searching for religious truth. I found a book titled, *When Bad Things Happen to Good People*, written in 1981 by Rabbi Harold Kushner, who needed to address the question of why in dedication to his son who died of a genetic disease. This is the kind of answer many people who experience illness or other tragedies are seeking. We all want the easy answers, but it's really the questions that are more valuable. Another book, *What Happens to Good People When bad Things Happen* by Robert A. Schuller, focuses on the Christian perspective of God as the dutiful, loving father. But even devout Christians might pause to ask, "Why did God let me get sick?"

There is no Christian doctrine saying that health and good fortune can be ensured in exchange for good deeds or being a good person. From a Christian perspective, a good life is not guaranteed on earth, but only in eternity. Another aspect of this perspective is the free will that God has granted to each of us. In this view, human suffering is like that of a child who hasn't learned a lesson. While God watches us as we learn lessons and truths, He hopes that people will make right — moral, ethical, and altruistic — decisions, so that each lost soul will come back to Him in the afterlife. Others might speak of our responsibility to end injustice and suffering, as God is waiting for people to spread love in the world.

Do you believe in God as a benevolent parent, watching over you and hoping you make the right choices? A God who wants peace, love, and happiness, who blames the Devil for the evil actions that occur in the world? Do you believe in a God of punishment, one who says, "I told you so but you didn't listen to me?" Do you believe in the bad luck of man falling prey to the natural laws of the universe? Do you believe there are bad people doing bad things, having a ricochet effect of bad luck on others? Lastly, do you believe that all mankind are sinners who should be grateful for the kindness bestowed on them by God?

From a spiritual perspective, if our soul remains constant throughout the universe, our time on earth is a short experience, and the struggle is the journey, filled with lessons we must learn to reach an enlightened self.

How can we bear pain, disappointment, or tragedy if we don't believe there is a purpose for our earthly existence? For many people who believe we are here for a reason – call it a spiritual contract if you want — finding meaning in our life makes bad experiences easier to bear. The reason may not be immediately obvious to us and we may not understand all the layers of cause and effect in the universe; in fact, the quest for this truth is often very long, but when we do find it, we gain a new and different perspective and clarity, which make our heavy burdens so much lighter.

Throughout history, people have tried to understand sickness from a combination of natural and spiritual perspectives. There are records from Neolithic times of the skull being chipped to allow evil spirits to be released and cure the patient of psychopathology. Even early Greek physicians focused on the natural imbalances of the body, but there were always diviners and priests ready to offer a spiritual explanation, and medicine was often offered in combination with a plea to the Gods. In China, medicinal drugs were used to treat diseases thought to be caused by angered spirits. Later, in the Middle Ages, people believed their illness was the divine punishment for their immoral conduct. Even in the modern world of science, the role of the placebo effect, the impact of individuals' beliefs, and mental fortitude have been studied.

I started telling people that getting a cancer diagnosis was the "kick in the pants" I needed to focus on true health. I didn't think of myself as a naughty disciple, but more of an adult experiencing light bulb clarities and forced to learn more about life and myself. This gave me an opportunity to dig deeper, look within myself, understand my psyche, be able to hold tight and let go and learn to be vulnerable. I was given a chance to grow, a chance to question, a chance to sit still, a chance to listen, and a chance to change. I didn't think prayer would work. Why should I ask God for help for something that was created within the chaos of Man and my own imbalances?

Researcher Valerie Curtis argues that "The history of ideas about disease… is neither entirely socially constructed nor a(n) 'heroic progress' of scientists leading the ignorant into the light and that we also have a biological nature to want good hygiene and avoid infection."[8] However, in our time the answer to why is different from what it was in the old days. We understand so much more about health and

---

8   Curtis, V. (2007). *Dirt, Disgust and disease: a natural history of hygiene*. Journal of Epidemiology & Community Health, Aug 61(8): 660-664.

our cells now than in the past, and it's hard to ignore this information and the power we have for healing.

Exploring a biological why is initially confusing. Of course, as soon as I was diagnosed, my first reaction was to Google possible causes. Cancer sites providing health information for Hairy Cell Leukemia mention that our understanding of how this disease develops is limited, but list these possible causes:

1) Exposure to radiation …. I have had the usual amount of dental and broken bone x-rays — could they have contributed to HCL?

2) Exposure to chemicals…. Does sniffing smelly markers in school count? What about cleaning my bathroom with a mix of bleach and cleaning solvents, creating a concoction of fumes?

3) Exposure to sawdust…. Okay – I was around my dad as a young child when he was building the house – did that count?

4) Ethnicity (Ashkenazi Jewish???)… Not me

5) Predominantly older men????... Definitely not me

What about Aspartame gum? I have a habit of swallowing gum, even though I know it is bad. Some people believe that swallowed gum will stay in our system for seven years as indigestible resins move through our digestive tract. Scientists tell us this is just a myth, but can I really be sure that toxicity of aspartame had not had any effect on my digestion, causing stress in other areas of the body?

What about eating unhealthy foods, even while exercising? When I finally started losing weight and was going to tons of workouts and boot camps each week, in the months prior to the diagnosis I wasn't always eating right. When I had a mental or hormonal low, I often ate lots of chocolate or a whole pint of ice cream. I would tell myself that I could start again the next day and work off the calories. But is it possible that in the meantime the toxins accumulated in my system? Was I actually able to sweat out and rid my body of these substances? Or was I creating chaos in my cells and then adding more stress because of the intense workouts and the release of free radicals?

What about not being my authentic self? I had recently left a job where I was making decisions that were going against my moral compass and exacerbating my history of people pleasing. From "looking like a good teacher" in Taiwan, where image is the first judgment of parents, to wanting to be a good wife, a good mother, and a good role model, I had spent more time waiting for the reassurance of a job well done and a pat on the back, than thinking about what reflected who I really was.

Cancer is not straightforward; finding health is not straightforward either.

My father died in 2001. I wasn't there and found out after he had already been admitted to the hospital. He died of a heart attack after the doctors had told my mother to go home, as she didn't need to worry that night. But he was diagnosed with prostate cancer that had probably spread. There were signs of illness several months prior, but no one mentioned cancer so it was probably easy to be in denial as he was getting things checked out. I think my mother once said that she had a feeling he was dying but never voiced that out loud because who wants that to be a reality? Meanwhile, his work and family commitments always took precedence.

Years ago – after my stint in South Korea as a backpacking ESL (English as a second language) teacher, I came back to a diagnosis of a breast cyst that turned out to be benign. I was keen to ask the doctor why I had developed this cyst, hoping that information would give me the power to prevent illness or answer my "why" questions. This was in 1996 and the doctor had no idea, saying that physicians didn't have an answer to why people developed benign breast cysts. I couldn't accept this and tried researching online. Alternative theories suggested that that breast tissue was connected to the liver. This made sense to me. I had spent the previous year drinking profuse amounts of Korean Soju (a harsh rice spirit and Korean's alcoholic drink of choice) and going through an emotional breakup. I got over the breakup, focused on less alcohol, and a year later the cyst was gone. When I asked the doctor again for answers, he said that he didn't know why a cyst disappears.

Q. Is it your fault or are you the victim of viruses and bacteria in your environment?

Several movies were made about a spread of infectious disease, such as "Outbreak" (1995) and I Am Legend (2007). I am thinking of the ones where the camera follows around an invisible main character; the airborne bacteria spreading from person to person as people hop on trains and buses, shake hands and cough in a shopping mall, unknowingly spreading disease. But what about a scene that is hidden and easy to ignore?

I believe we are influenced as much by internal bacteria as the external one. I am not a doctor, naturopath, face reader, or psychologist. But sometimes I have a whisper of a message about someone's state of health as it manifests itself in the body. It's a bit of a bad habit – when I sit at the coffee shop, I start looking at everyone coming in, trying to guess his or her situation… *Mr. A is close to senior and aging quickly. Coffee and sunglasses – he leaves a crumpled up paper on the table? Maybe he has inflammation and arthritis setting in as the immune system weakens. Mr. B sits with Ms. C close by. It's possibly a first date. They are both middle-aged. Mr. B has had too much sun over the years - he doesn't eat too much but is losing hair and muscle - possible stomach issues, as he doesn't like to deal with problems. Ms. C is aging well but her skin is dull – she didn't eat all her veggies as a young adult and focuses on being the perfect outer shell to find the perfect husband, pushing aside her true self to become the girl her mom wanted her to be. Mr. D waits for a drink at the cashier. Also middle-aged, he works out and has kept his muscle. Indulging in beers to relax, the eye-bags are growing. The stress shows on his face, as he doesn't know how to deal with ever-growing financial pressures. Mrs. E is behind him. She is a mom in a ponytail. She doesn't have time to focus on herself and spends a lot of time on her family and kids. She relaxes with a wine and some chocolate, telling herself that everyone has a bit of a muffin top and deserves to indulge once a day.* I am not keeping a secret journal and, yes, I did read *Harriet the Spy* as a child to warn me about not pre-judging people, but it's true that health and disease do show on the body. So while many people are looking at the outer and inner symptoms to diagnose our weaknesses, what if we could look even deeper and see what is happening in our cells and microbiome?

In *Gut,* author Giulia Enders, has a great analogy of our cell and bacteria universe by thinking of how the Earth looks from space. Observing the world from so far away, we can't see humans, even though we think of ourselves as an important part of the universe. Likewise, all our bacteria feel that they are significant as they roam around the brain in our gut, a very important organ. She states that we are influenced as much by internal as external bacteria.[9] This is a powerful statement of science, which means we need to protect ourselves not just from the germs outside; we must help create a good army of bacteria inside our bodies as well.

I tried to get a sense of this. If there are approximately 7.4 billion people in the world (2016 numbers) and each of us has about 30 trillion human cells, that means every individual has approximately 4000 times more cells in our body than there are people in the world and about 5200 times more bacteria in our body than there are people in the world. I had to spend some time figuring this out, and although these numbers are approximate, they are still overwhelming. It makes each one of us a significant macro-host, enlarging us beyond our concepts of "ants in the universe."

Q. Is it better to fight against whatever is making you sick or accept it? Or can you do both?

As I mentioned, I don't always respond well to the "fight cancer" slogans. However, I can relate to the concept of a fight going on within my body — that I am part of this battle, both consciously and unconsciously, and there is a whole host of characters in the fight within the universe that is my body.

When I go for a blood test, there is always a section that is checking my immune system, looking at neutrophils,

9   Enders, G., *Gut: The Inside Story of Our Body's Most underrated Organ* (Greystone Books, Ltd, 2015) p.266.

monocytes, leukocytes, and more; but I am not always sure what the numbers mean. I do know that these cells are trying to help me.

The neutrophils are white blood cells in the immune system that circulate around the body in the bloodstream. They are the first to begin killing invading microbes when an infection is sensed. They can release chemicals to destroy the bad cells or engulf pathogens with NETS — neutrophil extracellular traps — web-like structures that contain fibers to trap pathogens (this sounds like Spiderman)! After the attack, the pathogens have to be removed or some toxins might leak out, causing inflammation or infection. How does this happen? Cell death! The neutrophils are programmed to carry out apoptosis. It's like the ultimate suicide mission! "If a cell has undergone extensive oxidative damage, particularly to its DNA, the cell must either repair itself or, if the damage is too great, undergo apoptosis (cell suicide).[10] However, if they carry out apoptosis too early, they don't get all the bad cells and if they carry out apoptosis too late, some of the leaked toxins from bad cells can cause further infection… This is a lot going on!

There are other white blood cells called lymphocytes and there are different kinds of lymphocyte cells (T cells, Natural Killer cells, Cytotoxic T cells, for example) that are like soldiers in an army, each with specialized training, circulating around our body, scanning for infections and abnormal cells. Some T cells directly attack bacteria, viruses and cancer cells. Some recruit other immune cells. Some suppress the immune system to prevent over-reacting and others remember bad cells that have been seen before. Killer T cells are so

---

10   Alschuler, L.N. & Gazella, K.A., *The definitive Guide to Thriving After Cancer* (Ten Speed Press: Berkeley, 2013) p. 119.

specialized they could be said to have x-ray vision and can scan cells to spot problems.

I find it very encouraging that we have a system to fight pathogens. I somewhat knew this already but with a cancer diagnosis, it really feels like a war zone inside – and I want my warriors ready to fight whatever comes their way! When I was young, I wrote down a quote from children's author, Madeleine L'Engle, "In this body, in this town of Spirit, there is a little house shaped like a lotus, and in that house, there is a little space. There is as much in that little space within the heart as there is in the whole world outside." Her books had a profound impact on me as a pre-teen because they combined religion, spiritualism, and science in a way that seemed to constantly mirror life purposes and quests for enlightenment and love. One of the books, *A Wind in the Door* (part of the Wrinkle in Time series), so clearly illustrates the impact of what happens in our inner micro-biotic world. The main character is Meg and she is brought into a quest to help save the life of her brother, Charles Wallace. His farandolae (fictional symbiotic creatures inside the mitochondria) are dying, so his mitochondrion can't use enough oxygen. Meg's mission is to fight the "darkness," which are trying to keep the same farandolae from singing and joining other farandolae in their deeper purpose of life. Meanwhile, Meg's mother has coincidentally been studying farandolae and Charles is able to read Meg's thoughts and has an understanding of what's happening as he lies in his bed at home, struggling to breathe. In the events that unfold, time and space are relative and not important. His farandolae are dying, so his mitochondrion can't produce enough oxygen. "If the number of farandolae in any mitochondrion drops below a critical point, then hydrogen transport can't occur;

there isn't enough fuel, and the result is death through energy lack."[11] The author creates a universe of symbiotic connectedness from the atom to the macro and everything in-between. "That's how it is with human beings and mitochondria and farandolae – and our planet, too, I guess, and the solar system. We have to live together in – in harmony, or we won't live at all."[12] In the story, there are examples of characters (cells) who "exxed" themselves, rather than being taken over by the dark. This completely reminds me of the suicide mission of neutrophils.

Although fictional, these kinds of analogies between the micro and macro world and the synchronicity of life were mind-blowing concepts to me as a 12-year-old, and they still hold deep meaning to me as an adult. Listening to my gut, following a path of love, loving myself and giving my cells healthy nutrients can seem both egocentric and altruistic at the same time. But finding greater meaning for what is happening in my body makes me feel more connected to the universe. Focusing on "why" questions can also be an excuse for finding blame. This is a powerful statement because it means I can't spend time looking for the thing that caused my cancer. Finding blame isn't really possible and it also takes away from feelings of gratitude and looking within. I know it sounds crazy to think of being grateful for cancer and maybe it's easier to take this stance with a state of remission, but taking away the focus from finding blame makes it easier to change the "why me" questions into "how does my situation benefit me and others?"

---

11   L'Engle, M., *Wind in the Door* (Crosswicks Ltd: New York, 1973) p. 143.

12   L'Engle, M., *Wind in the Door* (Crosswicks Ltd: New York, 1973) p. 147.

Chapter 7.
G.E.A.R. up for life

When I tell people that I cured my cancer in five months, I feel obliged to continue the conversation with an add-on of how I did it. I am never certain how interested people really are to hear my story, so I quickly say that I did everything possible, using both standard and alternative treatments that I could find on the Internet. I wasn't going to completely ignore my oncologist, but I also felt compelled to find out my options for other support, searching for vitamins, antioxidants, and other healing modalities. I love the current studies in the field of epigenetics – understanding how we are a product of our genes, our behavior, and of our ancestors' behaviors.[13] I want to know more about how our environmental factors might not change our DNA but can affect our genetic traits.

In order to influence our health, we need to be aware of the systems of health that are being affected, not just organs and symptoms of disease. Inflammation, hormonal balance,

---

13   Enders, G., *Gut: The Inside Story of Our Body's Most underrated Organ* (Greystone Books, Ltd, 2015) p.145.

digestion, insulin functioning, and the immune system are huge parts of controlling our health. There are so many aspects to ourselves: the physical body, the mental body, the emotional body, and the energy body.

Q. How can you respond to the warning signs of ill health?

Get into G.E.A.R - *G is for "Heal your GUT"*

1. *Listen to your what your gut is telling you*

2. *Respect your gut microbiome*

3. *Include probiotics in your diet*

4. *Include prebiotics in your diet*

Ancient Greek physician Hippocrates (460-370 BC) is quoted to have said, "All diseases begin in the gut." Each person's gut health is different. Your gut bacteria is a product of your ancestors, your family's eating habits, and your own food conditioning. If you take your genetics and mess around with your bacteria, the result will be a storm in your gut! As integrative gastroenterologist and microbiome expert Robynne Chutkan noted, "Bacteria can turn on and off genes which means that if your predisposed to a certain disease, your genetic factors can be altered by your bacteria!"[14]

Chutkan also mentioned that paying attention to the probiotics and prebiotic aspect of food would improve your gut health. I am amazed at how important probiotics are for:

Suppression of pathogens;

---

14   Chutkan, R., *The Microbiome Solution: A Radical New Way to Heal Your Body from the Inside Out* (Penguin Random House: New York, 2015) p. 13.

Stimulation of the immune system;
Reduction of inflammation;
Destruction of toxins;
Production of essential vitamins; and
Improvement of the integrity of the gut lining."[15]

Getting your probiotics from natural sources ensures a multitude of strains of these healthy bacteria. You can try natural yogurts, kombuchas, Kim Chi, apple cider vinegar, or any fermented foods. There are lots of supplement probiotics available to us, but it's important to be aware of what strains we are getting.

Probiotics help keep our digestive system healthy by controlling the growth of harmful bacteria. Prebiotics, on the other hand, are foods that can change the bacterial composition of the gut. Since they come from complex carbohydrates, they don't digest as well and can ferment in the colon, providing bacteria which feed your microbes! Some examples of prebiotic food sources include: artichokes, asparagus, bananas, dandelion root, garlic, leeks, onions, radishes, tomatoes and carrots.

More importantly, your gut is the second brain in your body, telling you when something is wrong in your diet or your emotions. That's why the phrase "gut reaction" means "instinct" or "intuition" — that inner voice we all have but don't always listen to. Asking yourself, "Do I feel nervous or worried or insecure in my gut?" will serve you better than silencing your gut reactions with comfort foods or any other suppressive methods.

---

15   Chutkan, R., *The Microbiome Solution: A Radical New Way to Heal Your Body from the Inside Out* (Penguin Random House: New York, 2015) p. 168.

Get into G.E.A.R - *E is for "EAT whole foods"*

1. *Be aware of added sugar in your diet*
2. *Eat "clean" unprocessed foods*
3. *Be aware of the best detox elements for you*
4. *Eat healthy fats*

Now there's even more refined discussion about sugar – about how the pancreas can be affected as excess sugar raises insulin and converts sugar into fat being deposited in the liver. There have also been reports of negative changes in brain chemistry after just a few weeks of unhealthy eating.[16]

I love that all carbohydrates have the same molecular formula: $C_6H_{12}O_6$. It's just the formation that's different. There's fructose (from fruit sugars), which is used right away, and glucose (from vegetables), which is broken down into glycogen and used for energy. Now sucrose (refined table sugar) is made of fructose and glucose. So one could say it's the added fructose in the table sugar that's the problem.

If we reduce our extra sugar, then the sugar-craving microbes will be outnumbered. An easy gauge is to use a list of low-glycemic index foods as a reference. In some debates about sugar, the jury is still out as it's hard to isolate the evidence of sugar's effects on people's health over the years when there are other contributing factors from diet and the environment. Even with denials from the sugar companies regarding the detrimental effects of refined sugar, I know how I feel after eliminating sugar from my diet for a few days, how I feel when I eat a lot of sugar, and how hard it is to keep

16   Ross, A.P., Bartness, T.J., & Mielke, M.B. (2009) A high fructose diet impairs spatial memory in male rats. *Neurobiology of Learning and Memory*, Vol 92, Issue 3, 410-416. Retrieved January 30th, 2017 from www.sciencedirect.com.

it out of my diet. I don't need to wait for any more studies. This is not a new idea – even Jack LaLanne, the godfather of fitness in the 1950s, begged people not to have refined sugar.

Plants are powerful and not to be ignored but botanical medicine is not patentable so it's not as well advertised as other supplements and medicine. That's too bad because it's the easiest source of health. Some might argue with me, but I think it's also cheaper to buy a few greens than a bottle of soda. We need to eat for our cells, our gut, and our heart.

Farm-fresh fruits and vegetables (tomatoes –lycopene, vitamin A – beta-carotene, plus coffee, tea, wine- resveratrol, and chocolate-flavones) prevent or stop the oxidation (cell damage) of other molecules in the body.

Recently a family member asked me what is the value of antioxidants? The word became popular in the 1990s, but I don't think it's just a buzzword. They literally protect our cells naturally, without side effects. Oxidants are free radicals found in the environment (air pollution, cigarette smoke, UV rays, alcohol, and even intense physical exercise) and the body. They help fend off viruses and microbes but if you have too many, they can cause damage, leading to illnesses like cancer and heart disease. Some antioxidants suppress formation of free radicals, while others search for free radicals and remove them before they do damage.

In your body, oxygen is constantly involved in chemical reactions in cells where electrons are shifted around, removing electrons from sugars, fatty and amino acids, and adding them to other molecules like oxygen, to create energy. But this forms reactive, unstable particles known as free radicals that combine with other elements — the by-product of turning food into energy.

During chemotherapy, I was asked not to take any supplements, as they might interfere with the treatment. I didn't fully understand this but now I get that chemotherapy relies on the release of free radicals to attack the cancer cells and the supplements would have attacked those free radicals. One catch: if you take too many supplements, you might suppress your body's own ability to turn on its antioxidant defense system, which is why it's better to get them from natural sources like food.

I had a whole list of supplements of vitamins and minerals I was taking. Essentially there is not one magic list. There are lists of top antioxidant foods but if you are eating fruits, vegetables, and unprocessed foods, you can feel confident that you are targeting most of the top needs. It's like when you tell your children, "Eat foods with lots of different colors and you will get all the vitamins." Working with a nutritionist, you will be able to identify any specific needs for your body. If your body is very overloaded with toxins or inflammation, paying attention to how foods are combined can be helpful. Alkaline and starches can work together but if you combine acid and alkaline, they tend to neutralize each other, not leaving enough acidity to break down the proteins. Eating more mono meals (one type of food) and focusing on alkaline foods can also be beneficial. I like green juices to maximize vitamin and mineral intake.

Looking at the long list of vitamins I was taking during my detox after diagnosis and before I had the chemotherapy, it's hard to determine which vitamins were the most effective. There is a combination of the placebo effect as well. I still look for vitamin and herbal nutritional support but don't want to rely on them in place of whole foods. It depends on how well your body is absorbing the nutrients during digestion, what part of the world you live in, and the types of food you have available. I wanted to eat a lot of raw food for a while. But this works best in tropical climates, where it is warmer and lots of fresh fruit is available. Sitting on a beach in Thailand, I would love mangos, baby coconuts, and green papaya salad. In North America, I was often craving more warmth and fruits over winter, but these were imported or out of season. Following what is available in the climate you're living in is another way to benefit naturally throughout the seasons. As scientists study food and break down the nutrients, there are some who lean towards nootropics, or "brain food" that improves memory, focus, and mood. These are chemicals from foods that have been isolated as "functional foods" like cereals, bread, and beverages that are fortified with vitamins, some herbs, and nutraceuticals (believed to provide health benefits in addition to the basic nutritional value). In isolation, the nootropic supplements can act as a quick fix for helping memory, sleep, creativity, and willpower. Possible drawbacks of taking them are: 1) you lose a sense of relationship with real food; 2) you lose the mindfulness of gratitude for food; and 3) you lose the complexity of how food nourishes, interacts with the mind, and provides health in a multitude of ways, creating health or disease almost subconsciously while we go on with our daily lives.

There are a number of healthful diets out there. The phrase "flexitarian" was coined in the 1990s for a plant-diet, which includes occasional consumption of meat. Dr. Mark Hyman, founder and medical director of the UltraWellness Center, recommends a modified Paleo diet, which is based on nutrition that works with each individual's genetics. I also like Chutkan's term "Veleo," which emphasizes "a vegetable-based philosophy... where a limited amount of animal products is allowed but not required."[17] Struggling with leukemia, I needed the iron from protein but also had to make sure I ate it in small amounts and only the cleanest protein possible to not make digestion more difficult.

I am blood type O, which is traditionally the "hunter-gatherer" type, but when your immune system is compromised, meat products can take a lot of energy to break down, as well as eliminate any toxins or bacteria during digestion. When I was using a tracking app to monitor my food choices, the settings suggested 35% carbohydrates, 40% fats, and 25% protein. If carbohydrates include vegetables, fruits, and grains, I am happy to increase this to 80% with an emphasis on the low glycemic index foods like vegetables first. So my breakdown would look more like 80% alkaline and 20% fats (high quality) and protein.

Recently a friend of mine had a high ankle sprain and a broken bone. Surgery was suggested but since he was a borderline case, he decided against the operation, believing that leaving his body to heal naturally would be less invasive than planting screws and bolts into the bone, increasing the risk of arthritis or other complications later. He looked at bones as living and breathing tissue, instead of pieces of a skeleton that had to be put surgically together. Given the choices of powerful foods we can consume to lead our body towards healing, I believe this model of health can work. There is an often-used quote from an Ayurvedic Proverb: "When diet is wrong, medicine is of no use. When diet is correct, medicine is of no need." When I read this, I feel like I hold a potential treasure of power to create health in my body.

---

17   Chutkan, R., *The Microbiome Solution: A Radical New Way to Heal Your Body from the Inside Out* (Penguin Random House: New York, 2015) p. 124.

Get into G.E.A.R - *A is for "Focus your ATTITUDE for healing"*

1. *Believe you have the power to get well*

2. *Positively incorporate exercise into your life*

3. *Craft your reality*

4. *Work on your mind and heart*

Again, the power of epigenetics (biological mechanisms that modify the genetic code) comes up. You may feel like you're getting sick and the next day you either have a sore throat and stuffy nose or… nothing happens and you feel fine. What made the difference? Research, as well as anecdotal evidence, has shown time and again that there's a link between positive thinking and improved health. Can you feel hope? Positivity? Those of us who cope well with disease are said to be positive, optimistic, and not easily stressed. The opposite is the neurosis of fear – worrying about getting sick. This is like a self-fulfilling prophecy: chronic stress and anxiety can trigger health problems. I've found that looking within yourself to identify and accept your feelings is important —finding emotional health means being true to yourself. Picking an affirmation that works for your needs is also important. After all my medical healing, my newest affirmation to work on the self is, "I can find the wholeness of my soul and my authentic self in the universe by looking within." Say your affirmation out loud, in front of the mirror, every day.

Exercise is also not to be underrated. Releasing stress and dopamine are huge benefits when you're trying to get healthy. "Exercise also boosts the number of mitochondria – energy-producing powerhouses – in brain cells, theoretically helping to delay mental fatigue."[18]

---

18   Young, E., *Sane: How I Shaped up My Mind, Improved my Mental Strength and Found Calm* (Hodder & Stoughton, 2015) p.63.

Ultimately, hardships happen but you also get to be a participant in the script. Crafting our reality helps us set and achieve goals, and respond to life with the tone we set ourselves. I had a friend complaining about some of the complaints she was reading from her friends on Facebook. I pointed out that my Facebook didn't look like that because my friends were saying positive things! We have the power to choose how we see – and manage — our stresses, our challenges, and our environment.

Get into G.E.A.R - *R is for "Give your body the REST it needs"*

1. *Finding the balance*

2. *Creating space*

3. *Accepting the yin and yang (welcoming the light and dark, joy and sorry, comfort and chaos)*

4. *Letting your gut rest (fasting)*

I am a mom and I often need to remind myself how important it is to give myself as much energy as I give to my kids, my family, my house, my work, and everything else on the to-do list in my head. Sometimes it means scheduling exercise classes but other times it means finding a few moments to reset the brain. I have already been working on the physical, mental, and emotional aspects of my health. To bring back the energy, I realized I have to fit in self-care time There are many choices to be active in finding balance, including:

1) Progressive muscle relaxation

2) Deep breathing

3) Hypnosis

4) Meditation – creating automatic focus on the self and then letting go of the self

5) Guided imagery

It's not always easy to wake up earlier than everyone else to meditate when you've already gone to bed too late the night before, but on the days I do make the effort, I can really see a difference in my ability to step back and observe situations without reacting and immediately getting stressed.

Sometimes I can make do without the morning meditation session with a few moments of closing my eyes and breathing during the day, which brings me back to an energetic self and awareness of the present. I live in my head a lot — as well as living life, I am always analyzing or reflecting about the life I am living. There's a lot of mental work going on. So, giving my brain moments of space is like having the benefits of a quick nap. Focusing on breathing with my eyes closed, a song or a mantra for even one minute builds up mindfulness to recognize the random thoughts for their triviality. Mindfulness is a popular word right now. It comes across as less overwhelming than meditation. It gives us small moments during the day to stay in the present. With mindfulness, we can create balance in the brain, which is flooded by masses of information all the time, and create a pause so that we can respond and not knee-jerk react to the emotional stimulus around us. I can do this before getting out of the car to pick up the kids at school, before getting out of the car after running errand, or just after I've put the kids to bed.

My friend has an interesting habit of "hibernating." When he is overworked or trying to heal, he sleeps and sleeps, turning off the phone and computer, not being afraid to shut out the outside world to give his body a rest. With the pace of today's world and information being thrown at us, it's not easy to turn all that off when the body is shouting for rest.

I love the word "Dadirri." It's an Australian Aboriginal concept of deep inner listening and quiet, still awareness. By learning to listen profoundly we create a safe space for healing to happen. I don't really want nothingness all the time. It feels like I'm not participating in life and just watching from the outside. But jumping into the midst of all the drama that life can bring can be overwhelming. There is a great moment in the movie, Parenthood (with Steve Martin), where the father (Steve) is talking with his mother. In essence, she says that she prefers the rollercoaster to the merry-go-round, enjoying the ups and downs that life brings, rather than the security of the constant merry-go-round.

Fasting is a way of obtaining digestive rest. There are some studies of how fasting can eradicate cancer cells but the research is ongoing. It is logical to conclude that giving your body a break from inflammatory foods would encourage healing. When the body is busy fighting radical cells, it doesn't have the energy to expend on digesting large quantities of food. However a cancer patient isn't always absorbing the nutrients he or she needs from food, so taking away more calories might be risky. Each person needs to navigate his or her nutritional health carefully.

Being healthy is both easy and complicated. Curing cancer is definitely complicated. Some of the complexity comes from the fact that we don't control everything that happens in our body. There are hundreds of decisions made every day independently by millions of cells (the workers). I am the manager of my body but I need to trust that my workers are doing a good job without micromanaging their every move. When I was first diagnosed with cancer I spent hours on the

Internet, trying to find ways to control what was happening. On reflection, I think if I'm the manager of my body, I can create a good environment (food and gut health); set the tone (meditation, positivity, and energy of the spirit), as well as the pace (rest and restoration). If all these aspects are organized, my workers can do a great job of keeping me healthy!

Chapter 8.
Could I give up sugar?

When I decided to detox it was because I knew my history, how much sugar I have had. I was diagnosed with PCOS (polycystic ovary symptom) after I gave birth to my twins, increasing my chance of developing diabetes if I didn't make a change in my eating habits. I knew the risk was lessening after birth but probably wasn't completely gone. I also seemed to have a chronic acidity imbalance, not quite getting a yeast infection but always close. I needed to stay away from any excess sugar, no matter how small.

In my early teens, my mom told me that I was allergic to chocolate. I am not sure if that was really true, since most people would have an allergic reaction when eating excessive amounts of chocolate. On Easter and Halloween, I often heard the expression, "Just eat it all so it's gone." As children we might not have money for lots of meat or a variety of vegetables, but I remember filling up on sugar in so many different ways. I loved popsicles in the summer. We often had pancakes for dinner. When summer came and fruit was cheap, I remember the family eating a whole flat of strawberries and pretty much skipping dinner. Then there were the brown sugar sandwiches that took me until after University to wean myself off of. At Christmas there were caramelized potatoes and pickled red cabbage soaked in sugar. We used to make a Danish treat of rolled oats and icing sugar as the main ingredients after which we all seemed to take turns sneaking into the pantry to have a "kügler" out of the jars. When we visited my grandmother after school, the chocolate powder and milk were waiting for us, with the option of not having to mix the chocolate powder so that it was the last gooey syrup to eat after drinking the milk. Grandparents always had coffee time with treats. When I was in high school, I was part of the wind symphony. The reward for a good rehearsal was always a sugary muffin stop on the way home.

In contrast, my mom was a big promoter of reading cereal box labels so that we wouldn't be ingesting any BHA or BHT preservatives. We also thought we were doing a good job in avoiding extra fat by eating margarine instead of butter. We never had juice in the house and my mom made lemon sun tea in big jars in the summer. I guess the sugar moments stand out because they were connected to comfort in addition to being so addictive.

The timeline moves from the past to the present but sometimes the journey has not been straightforward. After remission, I got tired of constantly watching my food, scared to put anything carcinogenic into my mouth. After a year and a half, I felt I had regressed in the sense of using refined sugars for emotional eating and becoming physically less active; the brain fog also crept back in. It was time to wean myself off sugar! Starting the 30-day detox from refined sugars, high glycemic carbohydrates, and excess fructose showed me that this process was like going off drugs and so many of us share the struggle, even when our ultimate goal is to be healthy.

The following are my entries in my diary as I tried again to cut sugar out of my diet. I was inspired by my friend who had started a blog and was asking us what we were going to give up for the "No" in November, almost like a detox before the excess of Christmas. She had talked about giving up sugar and I was reminded that I needed to as well. What better time to start again than the day after Halloween?

November 1st, 2015 - Day 1

I've been here before… some say it's good to fail as it shows you all the wrong ways and gets you closer to the right way. Or something like that… Winston Churchill said that, "Success consists of going from failure to failure without loss of enthusiasm." Throughout history, there have been many people who failed numerous times before finding great successes: Thomas Edison who was told he wasn't smart enough to learn anything (and who famously said, "Our greatest weakness lies in giving up. The most certain way to succeed is always to try just one more time"); Walt Disney, whose first business sent him to bankruptcy; J.K. Rowling, who was once living on social welfare; Jim Carrey, who was once homeless; the list goes on. After seeing a Facebook meme, I recently started asking my children three questions: 1) How have you been kind today? 2) How have you been brave today? And 3) How have you failed today? I am not sure they love these questions but I'll keep asking. If I want to become a better person and contribute to this life, then I have to be willing to fail and keep trying. It's Day One of giving up refined sugars…. Again!

It's a bit of a déjà vu. I've done this before – sometimes successfully and sometimes I've barely lasted a day. I did it very well to detox after the cancer diagnosis, but at some

point, I always stop. I just told my husband about my plan
and suggested that it might be harder than giving up cigarettes. (He's on Day 10 of stopping smoking for the third
time in his life and says this is it now.) He nods his head
and doesn't disagree with me. I am surprised. He says he will
always miss smoking. I say I will miss the sugar too as it gave
me comfort.

Meanwhile, the irony is thick – I am having a leftover
pork chop for breakfast, as I don't trust myself to look around
the kitchen and risk grabbing the maple syrup or licking the
spoon of yogurt… My kids are having gluten-free pancakes
with syrup; their Halloween buckets full of candy and chocolate are sitting on the table with cartoon exclamation marks
around them.

They ask if they can have a piece of candy after breakfast
and I say yes. I finish my pork chop and try to decide if I am
still hungry. I am not but that's not the difficult part – I can
already feel my arms tingling and my head starting to spin
a bit. I am not sure if it's the detox from all the Halloween
chocolate I binged on last night as a final goodbye, or the
emotional effects of not having the usual carb load in the
morning, even it was just jam on whole wheat toast. I am
starting to stare out the window, concentrating on ignoring
what my brain is trying to tell me and warn my husband
that it's already hard. I hope I don't yell at anyone today. It's
not their fault – I have done this to myself and it's my own
journey… kind of. So, I decide breakfast is over, have some
vitamins that might help with the detox and start cleaning
the house to keep myself busy. Should I post on FB again?
Last time I thought it would help with accountability but
even the shame of admitting failure on FB didn't help. Wish
me luck!

November 2nd, 2015 - Day 2

I woke up this morning feeling better than I expected. No detox headaches or instant cravings as I had had the other times I've done this. So I started giving myself a little mental pat on the back and then realized, wait a minute – it's only Day 2!! It feels like forever already – like detoxing or giving something up or weaning off a drug. It feels weird to say this but I am a sugar addict! There are probably many of us out there who wouldn't give ourselves this label but that might be because the refined sugar is so prevalent in our foods. So many times my friends and family have said I am being too restrictive when I opt out of the foods containing sugar that are a normal fare for everyone else.

I remember the first time I tried to get refined sugar out of my cupboard. It was the beginning of University when I was easily influenced by books shaping identity and habits. I had just read the book, *Lick the Sugar Habit*.[19] Never before had I heard someone say that added refined sugar in our diet could be linked to a number of diseases including heart disease, diabetes, arthritis and even cancer. Back in the 1970s everyone was still talking about low fat, using margarine instead of butter, and worrying about cholesterol. But this book was saying the opposite! It linked the USDA's data on the average consumption of sugar (130 pounds per year) to causes of allergies, arthritis, heart disease, and cancer. It showed me how many red beets I would have to eat every day to equal the amount of extra refined sugar I was ingesting. The book was using data from the 1980s – by 2015 it was closer to 150 pounds per year. That's about three pounds of

---

19   Appleton, N. (1988). *Lick the Sugar Habit*. New York: Avery Publishing Group Inc.

sugar a week or 22 teaspoons a day — almost four times as much as we need. Imagine if I had listened then to what the book had to say – how would my life be different?

Everyday foods became red flags– cereals, bread, yogurts, granola bars, pasta sauces, canned peas, chips, ketchup, salad dressing... sugar was in everything I was picking up at the grocery store and the meats and vegetables were my only safe choices. I tried making my own granola with apple juice. I looked for low glycemic bread choices and started sharing my excitement about my new wisdom with my family. Well, you can guess their reaction. It's not much different from someone who has just discovered religion – that mix of superiority and confidence while trying to be genuine and excited. I read this book back in the 1980s while still a teenager, and my family thought I had gone extreme – everything in moderation was their response. It wasn't that I disagreed with them but something about what I had read was ringing so true to me – this was the missing link to health that I was looking for – the cure for headaches, hormone shifts, bad skin, weight gain, brain fog, itchy skin, and many other conditions. The question I asked myself was – what was the definition of moderation? Back to being a sugar addict...

November 3rd, 2015 - Day 3

I am struggling with the willpower versus addiction versus psychology of this whole process...

I am a smart, intuitive, creative, and kind person. Why would I struggle with giving up sugar? Does it mean I am just pretending to be strong on the outside but am actually weak on the inside? I am showing people that I've got it all together and then falter privately while listening to Sting's "Desert Rose," Adele's "Hello," or Sam Tsui's cover of "Don't Stop

Believing" over and over again. I take the last part back – listening to those songs while typing can be inspiring and puts me in a great mood. It doesn't match – being so strong and so weak at the same time. If I have a sugar addiction because of psychological reasons, there's lots of literature suggesting that my dependence is based on the feeling of comfort that sugary foods have given me throughout my life (no wonder we often use the expression "comfort foods"). As I mentioned before, when I was young it was all about the special food on special occasions. So much sneaking – shame associated with having treats but at the same time, a look of disbelief if you said no to the cookie offered to you: are you rejecting the love that I put into the baking? But is there a difference between eating the cupcakes that your grandmother lovingly baked for you versus a donut from Tim Horton's? Giving some reverence to the food should help: enjoying home-made foods rather than wolfing down a quick sugar fix from a drive-through, but does my gut know the difference? Science might say no but the "love of food" has a powerful effect. I was in Europe visiting my husband's family shortly after my initial recovery from the chemotherapy treatment. A beautiful cheesecake had been made for us. How could I say no without isolating myself from the group and disappointing my hostess? I love cheesecake but worried about breaking my resolve not to have sugar. But there was love in the dessert that had been prepared for me and it did feel different than sneaking a chocolate bar in the car when no one was looking.

There's another theory. Some research suggests that sugar addiction is a biological one that has little to do with my willpower, but is a sign of a strong survivor. In the days of hunting and gathering, finding a source of carbohydrates was rare – the odd fruit or berries. Evolutionary biologist,

Daniel Lieberman discusses how "millions of years of evolution favored ancestors who craved energy-rich foods, including simple carbohydrates like sugar that used to be rare, and who efficiently stored excess calories as fat."[20] So humans were attuned to searching this out and rewarding themselves when it was found. Hence the dopamine response: sugar goes in, the dopamine receptors open up, releasing dopamine and serotonin, the so-called "happy hormones" (other ones are endorphins.) So it is easy for the food to make us feel happy and explains why, when ingested on a regular basis, sugar creates an addiction so quickly: because it lowers the dopamine response until more sugar is required to get the same reaction. This sounds like a drug. In one French research project, researchers reported how rodents addicted to cocaine would choose sugar over the cocaine, leading to implications of the addictive potential of sugar.[21]

I remember being up and down emotionally when I first moved to Taiwan, no husband or kids, and searching for my identity while being surrounded by an adventure and surprises on a daily basis. Whenever you thought you knew what was going on, you didn't. But everything worked itself out. Eating out, parties, and crazy schedules affected the balance. After a few sugar-laden drinks or a dessert, I turned into a fun version of myself — Zena, as my friend lovingly called me. I didn't realize how unbalanced I was at the time. I thought it was my personality showing without inhibitions. The sugar high was a kick. I became creative — I could write

---

20   Lieberman, D. *The Story of the Human Body: Evolution, Health and Disease* (Random House: New York, 2015) p.16.

21   Lenoir, M., Serre, F., Cantin, L., Cantin, L., & Ahmed, S. (2007) Intense Sweetness Surpasses Cocaine Reward. *PLoS One* 2(8) Retrieved January 31st, 2017 from www.ncbi.nlm.nih.gov.

poems, paint, stay up all night, and discover the truths of life. Then I would crash and become depressed, or itchy, or get migraines and another version of myself would appear. Sometimes I would try to avoid sugar but it was hard when I needed to be polite in a culture that wasn't mine. When little glutinous rice desserts would be offered, the only solution was to say, "I am so sorry. I am allergic. The doctor told me I couldn't have sugar." Sometimes it worked. The thing is, when I avoided the sugar for an evening and had calm conversations around a dinner table, people missed Zena, wondering what happened to their fun friend. This wasn't fair –was I really more likable on a sugar high? When I was balanced, some of the creativity was lost. Maybe this is how it is for so many artists — there has to be a certain amount of angst and internal turmoil for them to be productive. In *10% Happier*, author Daniel Harris says that "equanimity is not the enemy of creativity,"[22] and that eventually taming the demons can make one more creative and becomes more satisfying than indulging the demons. I didn't want to spoil the creativity but needed to find health. This gave me some hope that I could have both. The neuroses were tricking me into believing that I needed them but they masked the true creativity that I could unlock with better health.

If I said yes to a healthier me, did that mean saying no to the creative and adventurous me? Would people still like me? Or could I be more and create more? All these questions just from a little piece of sugar…

22   Harris, D., *10% Happier: How I Tames the Voice in my Head, Reduced Stress Without Losing My Edge, And found Self-Help that Actually Works – A True Story* (Harper Collins: New York, 2014) p. 210.

November 4th, 2015 - Day 4

The Facebook status worked somewhat. The 10 "likes" meant that some people were watching my progress. If I failed, I wouldn't be able to be a role model for them or prove how much better life was without the sugar... and as a public failure, my self-esteem would drop. There are still the doubters – those who say you need sugar! Everyone ganged up on the Atkins diet in the early 2000's, promoting a ketogenic state of low carbs where you start burning your own fat for fuel. Nowadays, one of the front row books at the health food market is promoting a ketogenic diet recipe book! Low carb diets are viewed as Hollywood-style fads, promoting how to stay a size 0 and keep your energy! There are different expressions – I could say I am "eating clean," staying in the zone, cutting out junk, eating low carbs, eating less processed foods, eating more raw. They all get different reactions from people who think you're on to a new fad, which will pass. They are somewhat correct – but I am looking for people who agree with the seriousness of what I am trying to do, understand the difficulty of detox, and are ready to give me some supportive comments to keep me going.

The kids finished school early today. It was raining so I took them to the library before going home. The ice cream shop is right next door and they think library time means an automatic stop at the ice cream shop. I said, yes, but didn't want to stay in the shop. I held Kelli's ice cream in the car while she put her seat belt on and she was quick to comment, "Mommy, don't lick my ice cream. You said you can't have sugar, right?" Yes, Kelli, you're right... no ice cream licks, no sugar.

November 5th, 2015 - Day 5

Everything in moderation – I don't like this expression anymore. When people say this, it makes me feel like an extremist if I mention that I am working on not eating any refined sugar. It might have been more acceptable in the 1950s or 60s, before there was as much processed food as there is now, but it doesn't seem to work at present since "normal" for so many people is a ton of hidden refined sugars. Other people's idea of moderation is most likely in excess since there is so much added sugar in processed foods. People think they're doing well when they stop adding sugar to their coffee, not realizing that their cereal, bread, salad dressing, gluten-free cookies, yoghurt, pasta sauce, and coconut ice cream all have added sugar beyond the regular amount of glucose and fructose we get from daily vegetables, grains, and fruit alone. This is the first year, 2016, that federal health organizations have set guidelines about how much added refined sugars are appropriate. I am seeing numbers like 25-30 grams or 6-7 teaspoons recommended daily. I am also finding articles that have estimated the average at 19 teaspoons daily eight years ago! This means that the recommended daily amount is not "everything in moderation." It's really a shift down. It's more like detox!

I think I am doing okay – no headaches and not as many cravings as the first day but then again, I can't decide if I've cheated or not.

If I tested the leftover syrup on my child's plate of pancakes with my finger is that cheating? If I had pasta with the rest of the family is that cheating? If I had a cup of granola with almond milk after dinner is that cheating? If I added some honey mustard dressing to my veggies at lunch is that cheating? If I had one gluten-free, child-size pancake with my chia seed and almond milk for breakfast is that cheating? If I tasted the ketchup with a couple of my kids' French fries is that cheating? If the green juice that my husband bought is really a bunch of apples and kiwis with high fructose content is that cheating? If I drank the whole 300 grams of bottled carrot juice with 14 grams of sugar, is that cheating?

November 6th, 2015 - Day 6

It's not my family's fault. I have done this to myself and it's my own journey. Should all people stop ingesting sugar, or just those who, like me, have (or have had) cancer? When I share with friends and family that I am trying to do 30 days without added refined sugar, the reactions vary. They might be supportive, saying, "Go for it!" or "Good job! Others are less enthused, telling me that my goal is "impossible" or "quite drastic." Whether applauding or being judgmental, they tend to see my struggle to be sugar-free as an issue that doesn't concern them personally. I am thinking that my experience can show others what happens when you take out the sugar.

After watching "That Sugar Film," directed by Damon Gameau, it is impossible not to see how intrusive that substance has become in our everyday foods that many people think of as healthy. Even the makers of the film don't want to stop just at the documentary. Their website expands into action plans for children, more info, and a hope for educating others on the prevalence of sugar in our food. Watching a movie like this makes it impossible to ignore that this is an issue for everyone.

November 7th, 2015 – Day 7

We got my cousin to babysit tonight and I was excited to actually go to the city to see a Cirque du Soleil show. Before we moved back to Canada, Paddy and I didn't go on dates very often. Today it was raining but the show was amazing. When we got home, I craved a bowl of cereal. Why did I need carbohydrates and sugar after a lovely evening? Was it the glass of wine before the show that sparked a reckless feeling of wanting more? Or did it start a biological imbalance of craving more carbs? Did I have a feeling I was trying to suppress?

This often happens after I've put the kids to bed too. Dinner and bedtime and getting ready for the next day add up to several hours of me focusing on the children – their table manners, the mind games of picky eating, the home reading that needs to be done, the sibling fights when one is tired and the other one wants to tease, picking out books for bedtime reading, and having moments of life lessons to teach. It's all good but maybe my subconscious is overwhelmed. I am working at staying calm, patient, and being a good problem-solver, and all that is a bit draining. So after they've gone to bed, some feelings make their way to the surface. Dealing with these emerging emotions is another task on the already full "to-do" list, so having that bowl of cereal gives me a quick hit of calm and buys me a window of peace when time stops and everything is fine. That dopamine hit is like a drug. And just like for a drug addict it's never about the drugs, eating the sugar is never about the sugar, but about how it makes me feel or how it hides what I am feeling.

November 8th, 2015 – Day 8

Okay – so no one's really watching but me, so I am the only one asking myself if I have cheated? Some of the questionable items – antipasto, whole-wheat toast, processed Kim chi, pickled red cabbage, a store-bought fruit smoothie – they all sound relatively healthy but they all have added sucrose (is fructose and glucose combined). I don't benefit from the fructose. A piece of fruit a day is really all I can handle.

November 9th, 2015 – Day 9

I went to hypnotherapy for the first time yesterday. My initial intent was to ask the therapist to hypnotize me into having an aversion to sugar. My strategy was that if I could get enough days without craving sugar, then by the time the hypnosis wore off, I would have rid myself of the physical craving.

Unfortunately or fortunately, the hypnotist was not interested in short- term success. She wanted to dig deeper. I said I turned to sugar when I was stressed either consciously or unconsciously and she suggested focusing on what was making me stressed. Step 1: After moving from Macau back to Canada, I was still redefining and rediscovering who I was, while family and friends projected onto me their own ideas of who I used to be in prior years. This was causing me stress and disconnect. The hypnotist created a very helpful visualization of a bubble that I could create around me in social situations. In the bubble, I could define who I was without anyone else's expectations. I could also decide who I let into my protective bubble or how far they would be from me. It was kind of a social force field.

November 10th, 2015 – Day 10

So what happens when a friend or relative offers me dessert made for me as a token of love? Does it make a difference in how it's digested? Will it go down better because the food is being eaten in the atmosphere of love and a social dining experience? I think this is just wishful thinking because sugar is sugar and its effects are the same whether the treats were made with affection or not.

November 11th, 2015 – Day 11

A day of entertaining… here's the rub – I want to have people visit my home and have a welcoming, friendly experience. I thought lunch would be easier to prepare without having to worry about sugar and dessert. The menu included chicken and mango salad, Spanish potato tortilla, kale and red pepper salad, grape tomatoes, rolls (I wasn't going to have any)… so why was it necessary to make a zucchini loaf? I didn't have any and my friend didn't have any either! It sits there sending messages of, "Don't you love me?" Look at the effort that was put into making it – do I throw it away not caring about the sugar, or worry that I am wasting food and stick it in the freezer for some other guests?

Then came dinner. I was proud of my salmon burgers that were filling, tasty, and healthy with the exception of some added breadcrumbs. I ate the burger without the bun and added the side salad, and everything was all right. Then came the dessert that had been brought as a gift – Christmas cookies with sprinkles and chocolate brownie cookies with icing. I looked at them as if they were something from outer space. This was my best coping strategy. Try to associate highly laden sugar items with the idea of garbage, unhealthy foods, poison, etc. I have done this with one of the most popular soda/cola drinks (which shall remain nameless) and have ranked it way down as a choice, even below hard alcohol drinks. After watching YouTube clips of this drink being used to clean toilets and disintegrate teeth, it wasn't difficult to make a negative association with it.

This particular technique —negative association —works with treats to some extent. I think it is effective and then I realize I am adding other things like dates and carrot juice, and slowly working my way back to high fructose content with regular foods. It's all really natural, so how can it be bad? During the cancer detox, I tried following some of the vegans on the Internet who ate only fruits and vegetables. In order to get enough energy, they had to eat an enormous amount of fruit in the morning. They looked so healthy – one lady even said her eyes changed color. After two weeks of a solid effort, I wasn't hungry but I had gained about 5 pounds. I think the years of sugar had created PCOS symptoms and my internal environment couldn't handle too much fructose either. I had to cut back on all sugars.

November 12th, 2015 – Day 12

Only Day 12 but feeling better! More energy throughout the day – the afternoon slump is almost gone! It's easier to fall asleep. The nighttime or morning gas and stomach pains are gone.

November 13th, 2015 – Day 13

Today was a busy "helping the family" day. My sister and I were repainting my mother's kitchen. Knowing that I was going to be out for the day, I had to plan ahead. I didn't want to be tempted with sugar while in the midst of any potential family drama. I brought my own lunch, including some bell peppers for a snack. A day like that always takes longer than others and all of a sudden it was close to dinnertime. Soon the house was full and I took on the role of figuring out how to feed everyone. Why did I do that? I didn't need to have extra food in front of me that I wasn't going to eat. I guess I stepped into the older daughter role, wanting to help everyone. Old habits die-hard... but I didn't have any sugar.

November 14th, 2015 – Day 14

I think I need a support group, something similar to Alcoholics Anonymous, where everyone acknowledges that he or she is a sugar addict. The members would be able to understand the mental cravings mixed with sugar cravings that are hard to decipher individually. The group would be a safe place to share the struggle of giving up sugar in a sugar-loaded world.

November 15th, 2015 – Day 15

So close
Almost touching
Almost tingling
Almost feeling
Almost loving
And the moment passed
Almost thinking
Almost aching
Almost hurting
Almost feeling
It's almost gone again.
So close.

November 16th, 2015 - Day 16

I had another hypnotherapy session today. I am feeling strong and on the road to making progress. The hypnosis CDs seem to lessen the stress I've imposed on myself in lieu of real stress. I am taking care of the kids a lot on my own (my brother-in-law just died and my husband had to travel over for the funeral). It's getting dark and rainy and I still don't have many real friends, having moved back to Canada just a few months ago. On the flip side, I've told people I am writing a book, have hired a trainer for the 6 weeks before Christmas, and still getting renovations done on the house. The goal of hypnotherapy today is to meld the two parts of my personality together. One part of me wants to be healthy, be the best version of myself, contribute to society and not waste time. The other side wants to be creative, spontaneous, not have to micromanage everything and doesn't give a &$*# about eating healthy because sugar gives me a high so I can zone out for a while. I can see now that it's not really about the sugar. It's about finding out what drives me, what gives me energy, what gives me satisfaction, and what my authentic self looks like in action, without wondering about which side I am presenting.

November 17th, 2015 - Day 17

Paddy is going to Macau – he's packing and I am watching TV. I am feeling stressed but not sure why. Instead of relishing my feelings, I've gone to the front entrance where the last snack bag of Halloween candy has been sitting for two weeks waiting to be given away, as it's all candy that the kids don't like. I guess it's not my favorite either — it's full of gelatin and food coloring… but somehow I eat the whole bag, stuffing the empty bag behind the pillow as my husband comes in for a hug and kiss when the taxi arrives. How sad. Judging myself at the same time but can't stop this behavior.

November 18th, 2015 – Day 18

Somehow I've convinced myself that pure maple syrup is acceptable in the mornings, while the rest of the day is filled with lots of vegetables, fruits and low gluten carbs. This could be a slippery slope, though I have switched from mochas and chai tea lattes to plain lattes with soy and no sugar. Starbucks is losing its appeal without the fancy drinks.

I see a beautiful day before me but my
Heart is drowning in solitude, as my
Spirit tells me to dance joyously alone.
Freedom and quiet and choices abound yet
Today I can not feel what I know to be true.

Yesterday was so endless, each moment enjoyed.
Today I am lost and the moments are
Flattened by fear and thoughts of the future.
Why didn't I see what would happen?
It was only a bit of sweetness. Numbing the fear with
Subtle momentary pleasure
My body deceived me and said it would be okay.

Help me from drowning today. The light
Is missing from my eyes as I push a
Smile to my face. Everyone looks the same
But far away from my soul.
I'll reach out…
I know… sigh…. It's a beautiful day.

November 19th, 2015 - Day 19

Paddy and I went to a wedding today. It was a small gathering so everyone could sit around one table for lunch after the ceremony. We were the only guests invited who weren't family, so I felt honored. It was a beautiful ceremony and we enjoyed getting to know the family. I chose my lunch wisely and added a coffee instead of wine. But we all had set lunches that came with desserts. When it was my time to choose, I offered my dessert to be shared with someone else who wanted extra. I felt strong and told people I needed to keep away from sugar after surviving cancer. I don't have a good one-liner for these types of conversations to defend my actions. The only glitch was when I was sitting at the table, watching everyone else have the desserts, listening to the "oohs" and "aahs" and taste comparisons. Why do I need to feel so isolated when I am not participating in the sugar fest? I am old enough to march to my own drummer, but it's still nice to fit in.

November 20th, 2015 - Day 20

I am making an apple pie, watching myself put ingredients together, and at the same time, I'm asking myself, "Why am I doing this?" No one in the house is going to eat it except me and I am not supposed to be eating any sugar. We had lots of cooking apples from our backyard that I didn't want to waste and I had an extra pie shell from Thanksgiving that was taking up room in the freezer. Since it was just dessert, I shouldn't worry about wasting food but I convinced myself that was the reason I was baking it. The pie was made; I ate half. Then I felt crappy and threw the rest away. I am not sure what is the lesson here, except that it's obvious I haven't learned what I need to yet and the journey of self-discovery continues.

November 21st, 2015 - Day 21

It's getting close to Christmas, at least in terms of shops and sales. One of my sisters will be here to visit for the two weeks of Christmas break. This sets a timeline for my husband and me to finish renovations before she gets here so we can show her the house. But in the back of my head, I have another goal – I want to lose weight before she gets here. It seems it's a bit of a friendly competition but I am worried that the sibling rivalry might not be as harmless as we make it out to be. She's only two years younger so we grew up together and both struggled with weight and food issues. I used to be the one who weighed less than her and now the roles are reversed. Why does that bug me so much? I am all for goals and not eating sugar is helping me lose weight, but I want both my sister and me to reach our goals so that there isn't a winner and a loser.

November 22nd, 2015 – Day 22

Is the hypnotherapy not working, or am I overriding it? Or perhaps it's just too many steps forward and I am not ready? The maple syrup was a slippery slope… next was quick oats, brown sugar and almond milk as an evening snack, and then it was eating one of the Christmas cookies I was making for a caroling party. Next, I was eating a whole bag of caramel popcorn, trying hard not to read the label because then I'd realize that the first ingredient was sugar and not popcorn… I don't think I will make it to the end of the month.

I'm in a daze again
Everything around and around
Minutes and hours have passed again
I might as well be watching rain again

Who would believe the thoughts going round
The only thing to stop them is some music and some sound
The surrounding chaos prevent me from remembering
How simple it should be and the things that make me…me

November 23rd, 2015 – Day 23

Running strong with a drinking song in my head
Deciding, Duo, duality, multiple, split,
I need to be tough; I feel soft
I want to hold it in; I want to break free
I can handle things; I need to release
I want to take; I want to give
I want to fall; I want to be strong
Stay in the dark; reach for the light
Play the game or find some peace
Stop choosing and let it be.

I can't believe I wrote this a year and a half ago when I was dealing with cancer – having to fight and ask for help at the same time. But it's more than that – it's me, who's too complicated for her own good, boring everyone else. I don't need to choose – I just need to be me. Enjoy the light and keep it simple.

November 24th, 2015 - Day 24

I just had my final hypnotherapy session for the season. I expressed the frustration about two parts of my personality: 1) the creative side that wants to break free from rules, eat anything, party with lots of drinks, create art and poems and be spontaneous... and 2) the responsible side, which wants to set goals, live a long and healthy life, make good choices, and be the best version of myself. Once I was hypnotized, I could imagine myself walking down a path feeling light, feeling whole, and almost floating. I knew this was my true self. Then I came to a clearing and saw two women sitting on a bench. These were the two parts of my personality. I thought I was going to be asking the responsible one to let the creative one come out and play more. But as I watched them, I thought, "Why can't you two just get along?" and "This isn't the real me because the real me is already here." Amazing how the profound subconscious can send a message in the abstract. I enjoyed the session and thought it was enlightening. Yet, as soon as I got in my car to leave, the tears started — tears for my true self rightly seen and tears for my true self fragmented during so many years.

November 27th, 2015 - Day 27

So.... did I skip some days? I guess I could say I took two steps forward and one step back. I began the day having cereal with almond milk (it wasn't a kids' sugar cereal but a granola type that you think is healthy until you read the label and realize how high the carb content is). I thought I had a moment last night while scrolling on Facebook and saw someone post a blog about giving up sugar.... My computer cookies must be tracking me well. They said it was like an addiction and I could relate to this statement. We're not talking about craving something sweet after dinner. We're talking about everything in your brain telling you that if you have that dessert you'll feel so much better in every way and that you NEED it, and if you don't have it your brain will remind you after about two minutes that you REALLY NEED to have that dessert and that it's no big deal and that I should listen to my brain. Addiction, right? So this blogger said that what helped her cravings practically disappear was dill oil, Crazy, isn't it? I had heard about lacking calcium/magnesium or protein, or vitamin imbalance causing physical cravings but I'd never heard about dill. I thought it was maybe a sign for me to get back on track.

So I started out well – a shower, cereal, kids to school, went to choose paint for my bathroom wall project that day, and then decided to tackle groceries on the way home. I say tackle because I knew I would be bombarded by all the Christmas treats hype and chocolate sales. It's like an alcoholic walking into a liquor store — temptation is everywhere! I was doing all right until I wandered through the ice cream aisle. I saw Eggnog ice cream and thought, "Well, it's only available at Christmas, so maybe it's okay to try it," and then I saw hedgehog ice cream — a great blend of hazelnut and chocolate. I bought a pint of both and started to check out. As the cashier was ringing up my food, the previous customer looked at my items, saw the hedgehog ice cream and got really excited. "Is that hedgehog ice cream?" she asked as if I'd won the lottery. "Yup" I smiled back. The thing is… why were we having a sociable moment over ice cream? This is what happens with treats. Someone gives you homemade chocolate chip cookies and you thank them for being thoughtful and friendly, and then you both chuckle over how you both don't really need these sweets but you both agree it's the holiday season and it's ok to have sweets. So the only message I am getting is — if I give all this up, who am I alienating along the way? Sorry, I don't want to smile and say thank you for the cookies... no thanks, I don't want to join your coffee afternoon because there will be treats there that I will have to say no to. And how can I have people at a Christmas party and not put out some sugar? Ha ha – I just had a flash of putting out a bowl of sugar and some teaspoons, and tell everyone to help himself. I made it myself. Why hide it? Just put all the refined sugar you would eat anyway all in one bowl. You'll get the same high.

So what happened when I got home? I ate the whole pint of ice cream for lunch and passed out for an hour. No comment. No comeback. Just lots of haze.

Fragments of notes by my bedside
Pieces of unfinished art
Books that have been started in earnest
When things are halfway in between,
The potential seems most inspired
This is how it feels-
Cloudy and yet clear all at once
So much to offer yet nothings to say
I'm in the space between nothing and everything
Where dreams seem so wise
And beginnings are made
Thinking makes sense for a while

November 28th, 2015 - Day 28

I am climbing my way back to the surface again. I think it was self-sabotage or trying to escape… I've seen FB clips popping up that could give my struggle a name – how to be an introverted wife who wants to be there for the husband and kids but needs tons of time to recover from all the interaction. I don't want to live in my head all the time but I NEED it to let my brain process my day. I know it's just how I am and others are not like this but there are others who are. If J.K.Rowling, Bill Gates, and Mark Zuckerberg are reportedly introverted, I am not going to worry about this label. Another answer is "The Impostor Syndrome" — getting close to something that's new or creative that you are good at doing, but something stops you, perhaps a fear of being called out as a fraud? How can something creative and easy be worthwhile or called work? I was feeling the light and pushed it back down. Maybe I wasn't ready or maybe I was just scared.

Extraordinary in an ordinary world
I'm making my way
I'm playing ordinary
Surviving at the game
It seems a bit benign
So I push the limits
And my mind goes free
But it's hard to control
And I crash back down again
But who wants ordinary
I don't want to be the same
I fight my way back up again.
Playing extraordinary in an ordinary world.

November 29th, 2015 - Day 29

Is it the break in the weather and the sun coming out for a bit? Is it the cry I had, releasing tears of sadness for the self that has taken so long to blossom? I was wondering what kind of tears they were. I've seen pictures of various kinds of tears and it's amazing how different they are.

I am changing the playlist in my head again. Have you ever played the same song over and over again and drawn yourself into the depths of despair or the bliss of the moment? It can be all good or all bad. Is it perception? Is it blood chemistry? I had gluten-free pancakes with syrup, and orange and lemon juice with water; the fog is lifting but I've already cried twice. Is it blood sugar? Is it hormones? Exhausted adrenals? Too much living in my head?

I often tell people that the problem with reality is the lack of background music. Today it's "Alive" by Sia. Not bad for a life soundtrack.

November 30th, 2015 - Day 30

Have I been running away from acerbic tastes? Have I been holding on to the taste buds of a child, needing sweet for comfort? At university I used to identify with cereal and ice cream as foods I couldn't live without. I didn't see the craziness – I just went with the feeling... A post- breakfast snack needed cereal as a buffer for the day; an afternoon stress release could be found in a bowl of granola; dessert could easily be some quick oats and milk. Was sugar giving me more than a dopamine response all these years? Was it my anodyne to stress? Numbing the brain, ridding it of angst, giving an illusion of calm....

If I keep saying that I am a sugar addict, will it continue to have a grip on me? An astrologer would say a Gemini has a split personality. This used to be one of my stories... I need a dual personality... I'm a sugar addict... I'm a perfectionist... I'm a mother... I'm the oldest child... I come from Danish and German heritage...

Change your story... change your life. I am not sure who coined this phrase but I keep seeing it in memes everywhere.

I had a dream last night. My subconscious is definitely trying to send a message: standing inside and there's a knock at the door. I don't answer it and try to ignore it. But the knocking continues. It doesn't get louder but it doesn't go away. I am thinking, wait a minute – I am not ready. Let me be better – let me eat better – let me throw out this junk food. Just wait until the brain fog clears and I don't feel so sluggish. Just wait. The knocking continues. It's hard to ignore. I am feeling trapped. The potential on the other side is overwhelming. I am not sure I am ready. Quick, give me some carbs to hide behind for a while... to escape... It's a setup... for failure. If I open the door now, while I am not ready, I will fail and prove to myself I was right – see? I wasn't ready. If I don't open the door I will not progress and reach my potential. I have more to offer than living in my head. The energy is giving me a headache – splitting me in two again.

My head and heart say open the door but they also urge me to wait. I am almost ready. Time to follow my dharma.

Chapter 9.
Moving On

Cancer treatments are changing and evolving. Chemotherapy drugs usually target cancer cells that need to grow and divide but are often toxic to normal cells that also need to grow and divide. As studies are done to learn more about the differences between normal and cancerous cells, more effective treatment options could become available. I recently read a CBC news article about a study showing that bacteria was literally "carrying" chemo to the targeted cells.[23] I can't help picturing this as an animated cartoon. There's also continuing research on cancer vaccines. I hope more research also leads towards a melding of traditional and complementary or alternative therapies.

I was excited to reach a remission status. It felt like I had achieved my health goal. I still have blood tests every three months, but now I only see the oncologist twice a year. The remission status is great but it's so anticlimactic and not very final. Should I use the word survivor? Cured? Clear? If I still

23 Chung, E. (2016) *Bacteria coaxed to deliver chemo drugs right inside tumours.* CBC News: Technology & Science. Retrieved January 31st, 2017 from www.cbc.ca.

need to go for blood tests for the rest of my life, how do I keep myself from being paranoid about my health? The oncologists have implied that cancer could return in 10 years. I would love not to fixate on this, but I also like the idea of keeping tabs on my health. I should be lucky to have a blood test that shows how my health can be rated, though it's not showing any vitamin or mineral needs. It's not that easy to read a blood test. There are normal parameters given but the numbers used seem to vary by country, and I don't really know how to interpret the parameter measurements. What does it mean if my red cells are too high or my neutrophils are a bit low? It seems that the blood numbers are changing all the time too and everyone has different normal parameters. I like that I have copies of all my blood tests since I had been diagnosed and I can see where things improved, but the doctors don't have time to sit and explain to me what each section means.

I went to do a live blood analysis a few times at the local health food store. This kind of analysis is not very highly regarded among medical doctors. I am not sure why not. If the blood test readings that we have done are testing dead blood cells, why wouldn't it be more interesting to learn to evaluate live blood cells? From a quick prick on the finger, a blood sample is put under the microscope and looked at from the computer screen. I love seeing my cell activity at such a microscopic level. You can see if there are a lot of white cells; if there is inflammation around the cells; if there are bacteria growing; if there are immunity cells taking care of radical cells. I suppose there is some subjectivity to the analysis as everything is through observation and it is only a small sample of blood; however, my bone marrow test for Hairy Cell Leukemia was also confirmed by observation. It seems to me that the live blood analysis is less subjective if done by an experienced observer. Doing a follow-up of the live blood analysis keeps me motivated because I can see my cells looking healthy.

Now I am always thinking about my health – especially about obstacles to being healthy, such as too much added sugar in my diet. I constantly see it talked about in the media. For a while, it was thought that agave was better but now people are recognizing that it's close to high fructose corn syrup. Then there's the discussion of sugar alcohols like Mannitol and Sorbitol that are used as substitutes but tend to upset the bowels and not get rid of sugar cravings. I like stevia but only use it in my tea or coffee, or in the dried herb form on vegetables. Some of the brands of stevia have agave added to it so it becomes confusing for the consumer. A lot of health food stores offer Erythritol for baking but why not just avoid too many sweet desserts? It will be interesting to see how the mainstream diet changes as awareness of added sugar becomes more prominent in food marketing.

My next step is getting the kids off sugar. They barely eat any vegetables, so getting enough calories into them, never mind a variety of foods, is a constant issue that I hope they grow out of. I recently stopped giving them juice during the day except for at breakfast. Eliminating sugar should be a simple process but it is found in so many foods they eat — like granola and spaghetti Bolognese with ketchup, crackers, and yogurt with syrup, etc. — that getting totally rid of it seems almost impossible. Instead of being addicted to sugar, I am becoming addicted to quitting sugar. Instead of binging on bad foods and then going on extreme diets, I am finding a balance. Instead of working until burnout, I am kind to myself when rest is needed. The doctors use the word "remission," but I feel cured.

This is my own journey but I love having people around me to support me. My kids are a great example of this.

> Facebook 5:48 am ... my alarm had gone off a few minutes before. My daughter wakes up (in bed next to me after a nightmare a few hours before) and says, "Mommy, what about your exercise?"... Yes, thanks Kelli, I'm up now. #familysupport #thrivingnotsurviving

I hope that as I surround myself with people who are motivating me to be my best, I can encourage others to not give up and be their best as well. I also want to send this message to my kids and be a positive role model for them.

I often wonder whether or not I should tell people I am a cancer survivor. Should I remove the label? Do I even want a label? It's certainly not all that I am. When I moved with my husband from Taiwan to Macau, we had a funny conversation where I suggested he had an opportunity to color his hair. He had recently gone completely gray and I thought since no one knew him in Macau, he could cover the gray and start a new look! As his hair was so short, we quickly realized that he would have to color it every couple of weeks to hide the gray roots and decided against the idea. But changing countries can give you a fresh start. So when we moved back to Canada, I had a moment of trying to decide whether or not I should tell people I had cancer. I weighed a lot less than I used to, and I also had a completely different perspective than I used to. Did people need to know the old me or could we just start afresh? Sometimes people don't want to hear about someone's aches and pains. My grandmother always thought it was funny when people in shops asked her how she was doing that day. She knew they didn't really want to know, so she chose not tell them about her problems or worries of the day. But if you have a scar and someone else has the same scar, it often helps him or her to hear how you got your scar. Sharing your story so that the other person knows that you've experienced a similar pain has value. Having had cancer doesn't define me but it has greatly impacted my life. Cancer has led me onto a fast-track quest to find better health.

Q. Do you believe you have a future of struggling against disease or a future of experiencing vibrant health?

Everyone deserves to find their authentic self… their true health… I already mentioned that I am grateful. People look at me strangely when I say I am grateful for getting cancer. Maybe it's flippant to be grateful when I recovered so quickly, knowing that others struggle for years. Hippocrates said, "Healing is a matter of time, but it is sometimes also a matter of opportunity." I'm so thankful for a journey that leads me to a better version of myself. I recently watched Jane Fonda on a TEDx presentation for women. She envisioned a new model of aging. Instead of an arch where we peak at middle age and then end in decline, she sees a staircase where we can reflect and find ourselves as we mature. I like the idea that we are all struggling to become better versions of ourselves, improving the universe with each dancing soul. When I think of beauty, I am trying to look past the weight loss, past the muscles, and past the transformation. Instead, I am striving to like the person that is being reflected back to me and to identify with the beauty of strength of someone who is willing to continue the journey.

There were a few years while I was reaching the end of my 20s when moving to Southeast Asia had a profound effect on my life. Prior to this move, I was fitting myself into the role of a teacher, a potential wife, and what I thought was a good person. I enjoyed music, creativity, and finding moments of philosophical pondering. But I also craved a certainty to life, believing that if I did what I thought was the right thing, I would not only find my path but also create harmony in the universe that would be reflected back to me by a cocoon of security. Moving to Southeast Asia showed me the beauty of chaos and adventure and being in the moment to enjoy whatever was going to come my way. Then there was a huge earthquake resulting in years of panic and anxiety because I felt powerless in my actions to prevent a sudden disaster. My cocoon couldn't protect me anymore. Later, when I had children, I wanted to give them routine, security, and protection … pushing away some of the potential moments of spontaneity because they brought chaos and potential uncertainty. As the years went on, I thought I still needed certainty. It's not really possible. Change is the only constant, whether it's positive or negative. Author, Dr. William Hablitzel, has come to understand the benefit of this constant after spending years with patients who had devastating medical challenges:

"I have come to see opportunity as a friend, the type of friend who is willing to anger you in the effort to help you. Oddly enough, it is the last piece of the puzzle. For some it is the most important piece, as it forces us to spend time in the present moment. No one is promised a tomorrow, and in the moment we recognize that, we find ourselves in the present moment – the time for miracles, gratitude, service and happiness."[24]

---

24   Hablitzel, W.E., M.D. *Dying was the Best Thing That Ever Happened to Me.* (Austin: Sunshine Ridge Publishing, 2006) p.232.

Imagine a selection of parallel universes. Now imagine that you can step across to a different reality. Sometimes it's just a small shift, but looking at this possible new self from the outside gives us an enlightened perspective. Now we can give ourselves permission to step outside our current label, circumstance, projection, or expectation, and create a new reality.

So I began this journey from a perspective of surviving cancer. I wanted to promote the benefits of taking out sugar, processed food, and toxins. As I continued to keep a journal, the journey of writing and reflecting took me to awareness of how it felt to take control of my health, and made me want to share with others how much was possible – to not be a victim, to not take a passive role, and not to blame others for your misfortunes. I wanted to find my true self that was hiding behind stress-eating, misplaced expectations, and labels that I felt were covering my potential to thrive. Moving forward, it's not really about cancer. Bad things (or perceived bad things) happen to each one of us. Some people are ready to attack the bad things that happen to them by saying, "You're not going to break me. I am stronger than whatever life throws at me." Yet an even stronger catalyst is the hope that whatever brings us down in life, the human spirit can still rise. Everyone has a choice of how to respond to events that happen. When I was ordered to go on 12 weeks of bed rest for my pregnancy, every day was a struggle. I started looking up comments and chat groups from other people who were on bed rest longer than I was. There was always someone worse off or with a sadder story to be found. It told me that if someone else can make it through, so can I. I needed the push to focus on my spirit and being positive. I did the same thing when I was diagnosed with cancer. It is the only choice - move forward, choose love, let your soul shine through, and find your own health.

Recommended reading and viewing:

Books:

Lick the Sugar Habit
10% Happier
Heal the Gut
Book about mom and family giving up fructose for a year
Gut: The Inside Story of Our Body's Most Underrated Organ
The Microbiome Solution: A Radical New Way to Heal Your
    Body from the Inside Out
The Story of the Human Body: Evolution, Health and Disease
The Case Against Sugar

Film:

Forks over Knives
Food Matters
Sugar Coated
Fat, Sick and Nearly Dead
Crazy Sexy Cancer
That Sugar Film
Ted Ex video explaining sugar –
John Yudkin – Pure, White and Deadly 1969

Health advocates:

David Gillespie
Lo Han
David Wolfe
Dr. Rustig Lustig
Michael Pollan
Dr. Mark Hyman

Kris Carr
Chris Wark
Chris Kresser
Gary Taubes
Dan Beuttner

Follow Gina on her journey:

gina@findingmyhealthy.com

facebook.com/ginafindingmyhealthy